T0074334

MEDICAL RADIOLOGY

Radiation Oncology

Editors:
L. W. Brady, Philadelphia
H.-P. Heilmann, Hamburg
M. Molls, Munich
C. Nieder, Bodø

B. Jeremić · S. Pitz (Eds.)

Primary Optic Nerve Sheath Meningioma

With Contributions by

G. Bednarz · M. Buchgeister · E. B. Butler · S. T. Chao · J. O. Hernandez · J. Hinojosa
B. Jeremić · J. S. Kennerdell · D. Linero · S. S. Lo · M. F. Mafee · J. H. Naheedy
A. C. Paulino · F. Paulsen · S. Pitz · G. Reifenberger · M. J. Riemenschneider · J. H. Suh
B. S. Teh · R. E. Turbin · S. Villà · M. Werner-Wasik · H. Wilhelm

Foreword by

L. W. Brady, H.-P. Heilmann, M. Molls, and C. Nieder

With 102 Figures in 134 Separate Illustrations

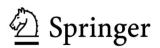 Springer

Branislav Jeremić, MD, PhD
International Atomic Energy Agency
Wagramer Strasse 5
P.O. Box 100
1400 Vienna
Austria

Susanne Pitz, MD, PhD
University Eye Hospital
Langenbeckstrasse 1
55101 Mainz
Germany

Medical Radiology · Diagnostic Imaging and Radiation Oncology
Series Editors:
A.L. Baert · L.W. Brady · H.-P. Heilmann · M. Knauth · M. Molls · C. Nieder · K. Sartor

Continuation of Handbuch der medizinischen Radiologie
                 Encyclopedia of Medical Radiology

ISBN 978-3-540-77557-7   e-ISBN 978-3-540-77558-4

DOI 10.1007/978-3-540-77558-4

Library of Congress Control Number: 2008925011

© 2008 Springer-Verlag Berlin Heidelberg

Cover design: Frido Steinen-Broo, eStudio Calamar, Spain
Production, reproduction and typesetting: le-tex publishing services oHG, Leipzig, Germany

Printed on acid-free paper

9 8 7 6 5 4 3 2 1

springer.com

DEDICATION

To my wife Aleksandra and my daughter Marta, for their endless encouragement and support during this project and throughout my career.
B. Jeremić

Für Andreas
S. Pitz

Foreword

Optic nerve sheath meningiomas represent a rare tumor about which very little has been published in the literature over the last 50 years. Therefore, there remains a major lack of information relating to the disease process and how best to treat such tumors. These tumors can arise intraorbitally, intracanalicularly, or intracranially. In general, they proceed by local continuous extension along the optic canal into the orbit or into the base of the brain.

This book — put together by Professor Branislav Jeremić and Professor Susanne Pitz — covers all the important aspects of the diagnosis and treatment of this disease process. The authors represent experts in the field relative to this disease process and their recommendations relative to general considerations, clinical presentation, the necessary clinical examinations, and techniques for diagnosis with imaging and histology are very appropriately and properly presented.

From these data, treatment options can be developed that allow for surgical intervention or external beam radiation therapy or stereotactic fractionated radiation therapy using the newest of technologies available in radiation oncology.

Aggressive intervention and appropriate proper treatment are associated with good results relative to management, and emerging from these discussions is the fact that the majority of patients can be treated adequately and appropriately with the newest technologies in radiation oncology.

The work presented by Professors Jeremić and Pitz represent a significant and important documentation of the approach to treatment in this disease process.

Philadelphia	Luther W. Brady
Hamburg	Hans-Peter Heilmann
Munich	Michael Molls
Bodø	Carsten Nieder

Preface

As an extremely rare and benign disease with virtually no lethal outcomes, optic nerve sheath meningioma has traditionally been treated worldwide with different approaches, and without a consensus on both how to diagnose and treat it. With only occasional reports in the literature, and with those reports being predominantly single-institutional experiences with few anecdotal cases discussed, optic nerve sheath meningioma remains on the fringes of oncological "happenings" and is rarely covered by the media.

Why then write a book about it?

Because time has come to begin a new chapter in this story. Many years have been spent improving our clinical understanding of the disease, our ability to diagnose it better and the treatments available to patients. These developments have led to a shift in treatment towards non-surgical options, primarily radiotherapy. With the safer and more precise use of CT and/or MRI, and the development of computer-driven treatment planning and execution, radiotherapy has become capable of delivering adequate doses to the tumor with minimal surrounding/safety margins, which has led to lower toxicity. The most recent results obtained with stereotactic fractionated radiation therapy indicates that a change in the existing practice in a majority of patients is needed.

This book is a summary of what we have learned and what we know today. It also represents a comprehensive guide to the most important aspects of the diagnosis and treatment of the disease.

A distinguished group of optic nerve sheath meningioma experts have contributed to this book. These colleagues have spent their professional lives dedicated to better understanding and treating this disease, and have made substantial contributions to the field in recent decades. With their work and dedication, we have been able to create a book that presents the current state of the art in the field of diagnosis and treatment of optic nerve sheath meningioma, and the effort should lead to a more optimized and individualized approach in patients with this disease.

We would like to thank all of our former and current colleagues with whom we have collaborated during the past decade. Their tireless efforts and dedication to the cause has made our professional lives more interesting and rewarding.

We would also like to express our thanks to the Alexander von Humboldt Foundation, Bonn, for its continuous support of B. Jeremić since 1998. Special thanks to Ms. Ursula Davis and Ms. Anne Strohbach for their kind, patient, flexible and effective management during the preparation of this book. Without them, the book would not have been possible.

Vienna
Mainz

BRANISLAV JEREMIĆ
SUSANNE PITZ

Contents

Overall Introduction, Problem Definition, Incidence

Branislav Jeremić and Susanne Pitz

CONTENTS

> ### KEY POINTS
>
> ONSM is a rare tumour. It is usually separated into the primary ONSM (pONSM) (intraorbital or intracanalicular) and secondary (sONSM) (intracranial). The tumour can also originate within the optic nerve sheath in the orbit or optic canal and may grow intracranially to involve various structures there. ONSM can also present in a bilateral form. pONSM represent approximately 96% of all intraorbital and approximately 1%–2% of all intracranial meningiomas. It is the second most common orbital tumour after optic nerve gliomas, but represents only 10% of all ONSM, all the others (90%) being secondary ONSM. Of the pONSM, approximately 96% are true pONSM and only 4% were considered ectopic; pONSM typically develop in middle aged women with the proportion of females ranging from 70 to 80, although they do occur in children as well.

1.1

Introduction

Optic nerve sheath meningioma (ONSM) is a rare tumour. It is usually separated into the primary ONSM (pONSM) which arise from the cap cells of the arachnoid surrounding the intraorbital (Figs. 1.1–1.3) or, less commonly, the intracanalicular portions of the optic nerve (Figs. 1.4–1.7), and secondary (sONSM), which arise intracranially, usually from the sphenoid ridge or tuberculum sellae and subsequently invade the optic canal and orbit by extending between the dura and arachnoid of the optic nerve in these regions. The term ONSM thus does not imply a definite site of origin. Nevertheless, once this type of tumour gains access to the subdural space of the intracanalicular or intraorbital optic nerve, the tumour grows up and down the sheath, invading the dura and obliterating the pial blood supply. In most instances, the tumour encircles the optic nerve without invading it. In other cases, the tumour may invade the nerve by growing along the fibrovascular septa (Samples et al. 1983; Probst et al. 1985). Such a tumour may eventually surround and obstruct the central retinal vein, central retinal artery, or both

B. Jeremić, MD, PhD
International Atomic Energy Agency, Wagramer Strasse 5, P.O. Box 100, 1400 Vienna, Austria

S. Pitz, MD, PhD
University Eye Hospital, Langenbeckstrasse 1, 55101 Mainz, Germany

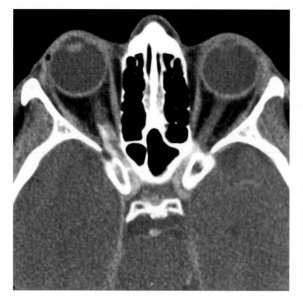

Fig. 1.1. Axial, contrast enhanced CT with demarcation of the (primarily calcified) tram-track-like tumor in the precanalicular part of the right intraorbital optic nerve

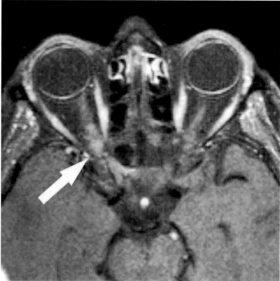

Fig. 1.2. Corresponding axial T1-weighted (T1w), contrast enhanced, fat-supressed view with signal, enhancement of the tumor (*white arrow*)

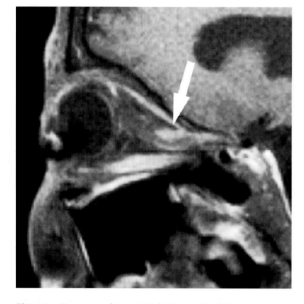

Fig. 1.3. Corresponding sagittal T1-weighted (T1w), contrast enhanced, fat-supressed view with signal enhancement of the tumor (*white arrow*)

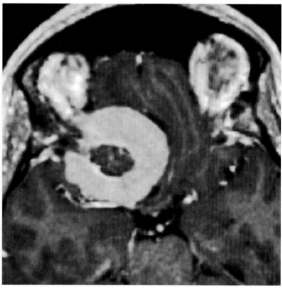

Fig. 1.4. Axial T1w, contrast-enhanced view at the level of the clinoid process

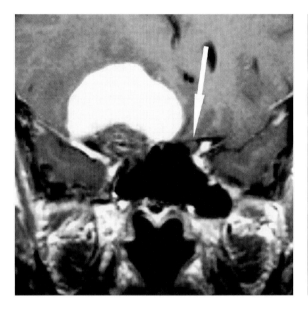

Fig. 1.5. Coronal T1w, contrast enhanced view at the level of the optic canal. No differentiation of the right optic nerve due to tumor compression. Note the corresponding left optic nerve in the optic canal (*white arrow*)

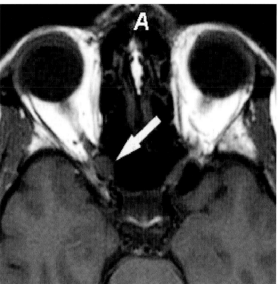

Fig. 1.6. Axial T1w, native view of the intracanalicular part of the optic nerve demonstrating a slight enlargement

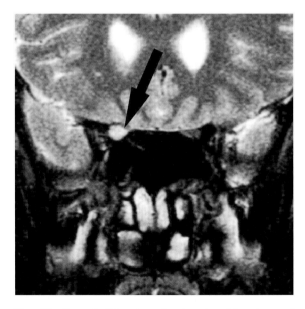

Fig. 1.7. Coronal, T2w view, showing the dislocation and compression of the right optic nerve (*black arrow*) by the inferiorly excentric (hyperintense) meningeoma

vessels. Rarely, a tumour will break through the dural sheath of the optic nerve to invade other orbital structures. Finally, a tumour that originates within the optic nerve sheath in the orbit or optic canal may grow intracranially to involve the optic chiasm, contralateral optic nerve, and internal carotid artery. It may even invade the cavernous sinus or the sella turcica.

ONSM can also present in a bilateral form (DANDY 1922; CRAIG and GOGELA 1949; SALAZAR et al. 1977; HOLLENHURST et al. 1977; TROBE et al. 1978; HART et al. 1980; WILSON 1981; COHN 1983), featuring invasion of both optic canals by one or several meningiomas. In some cases extended periods of time separating the involvement of the first eye from that of the second have been reported, casting some doubt on the causes of visual loss in the first eye (TROBE et al. 1978). Other authors (HART et al. 1980) suggested that the tumour may in fact have arisen multifocally, simultaneously involving both optic nerves in their intraorbital and intracanicular portions. The near simultaneous involvement of both optic nerves and the symmetric clinical course, accompanied by the surgical finding of an absence of tumour within the prechiasmal space, supports this conclusion (HART et al. 1980).

Although these (ONSM) tumours are frequently discussed together, due to different clinical characteristics, treatment, and outcome, all of which may have implications for the future strategies; they will *not* be discussed together in this book. This book focuses on the primary ONSM, in which both intraorbital and intracanalicular ONSM will be placed. The aim of this book is to summarize pretreatment and treatment characteristics of pONSM, putting a special emphasis on the use of external beam radiation therapy (RT) in the management of this disease, in particular stereotactic fractionated radiation therapy (SFRT).

1.2 Incidence

There has been some controversy regarding the incidence of pONSM because of their infrequent occurrence, the difficulty of determining the actual site of origin of large tumours (SPENCER 1972; ALPER 1981) and the possible confusion between meningiomas and the arachnoid hyperplasia that often accompanies optic gliomas (COOLING and WRIGHT 1979). In the Harvey Cushing's series of 313 meningiomas (CUSHING and EISENHARDT 1938), there was only one which arose from the sheath of the optic nerve. Other series of both meningiomas and orbital tumours support this rarity; various series have shown their incidence to vary between 2% and 6% (CRAIG and GOGELA 1949; DANDY 1941; INGALLS 1953; SHIELDS et al. 2004). In addition, the majority of the data come from ophthalmological literature (CRAIG and GOGELA 1949; KARP et al. 1974; WRIGHT 1977; MARK et al. 1978; ALPER 1981; SAMPLES et al. 1983), which may not be easily available to physicians from other specialties.

It is now established that primary ONSM represent approximately 96% of all intraorbital and approximately 1%–2% of all intracranial meningiomas (DUTTON 1992). It thus is the second most common orbital tumour, after optic nerve gliomas (CRAIG and GOGELA 1949; D'ALENA 1964; WRIGHT et al. 1980; SIBONY et al. 1984; ROOTMAN 1988; GABIBOV et al. 1988; DUTTON 1992). However, it represents only 10% of all ONSM, all other (90%) being the secondary ONSM. Of the pONSM, it is said that approximately 96% are true pONSM and only 4% were considered ectopic, i.e. those arising from ectopic arachnoid cells within the orbital

interstitial tissues or along the orbital nerves (CRAIG and GOGELA 1949; ROOTMAN 1988). These ectopic, extradural meningiomas do not appear to have a connection to the optic sheath or the optic canal and do not have an intracranial origin. They probably arise from congenitally displaced nests of meningothelial cells along the orbital wall or within the muscle cone and have been named "extradural orbital meningioma" (CRAIG and GOGELA 1949; ALPER 1981). Of all pONSMs, 92% arise intraorbitally and only 8% intracanalicularly (DUTTON 1992). Most of these tumours are unilateral, with 5% presenting bilaterally. They typically affect middle-aged women. There is no strong evidence for predilection for left or right laterality (DUTTON 1992). Interestingly, canalicular meningiomas had a higher incidence of bilaterality (38%) than ONSMs within the orbit (DUTTON 1992). In a subsequent series (SAEED et al. 2003), half of the patients with bilateral ONSMs had tumours along the planum sphenoidale in continuity with the lesions in both optic canals. Thus, it would appear that some cases of apparently bilateral ONSMs are truly bilateral, whereas others represent either the spread of a planum sphenoidale meningioma to both optic canals or of a unilateral ONSM across the planum to the contralateral optic canal.

Recent study from Denmark (LINDEGAARD et al. 2002) showed that frequency of ONSM increased significantly during the last 25 years. A significant difference in the mean ages of men and women with ONSM was found ($p < 0.05$, Student's t-test). The mean age for women was calculated at 48.8 years, being higher than the mean age calculated in the series of DUTTON (1992) (40.8 years) both being higher than that for men, calculated at 29.7 years in the Danish study (LINDEGAARD et al. 2002). This increase in incidence may have been the result of the development of better imaging techniques for investigation of lesions involving the optic nerve which became available in the recent years. However, in the same time period there was no significant increase in the incidence of malignant tumours invading the optic nerve, challenging improvement in imaging as the likely reason for such an increase in the incidence of optic nerve sheath meningiomas. The reasons for this increase, therefore, remain currently unknown; however it may reflect an overall increase of meningiomas which has been otherwise reported from Scandinavia, but not for other European countries (LOUIS et al. 2007).

As with other meningiomas, pONSM typically develop in middle-aged women (WRIGHT 1977; WRIGHT et al. 1980; ALPER 1981; SIBONY et al. 1984), with remarkably consistent gender ratio with the proportion of females in several series ranging from 70% to 80%

(CRAIG and GOGELA 1949; KARP et al. 1974; REESE 1976; WRIGHT 1977; WRIGHT et al. 1980; ALPER 1981; SIBONY et al. 1984). Nonetheless, they do occur in children as well. VALLAT et al. (1981) described a 2-year old girl in whom such a tumour occurred, and other investigators have described similar cases (DANDY 1941; OFFRET 1951; DUNN and WALSH 1956). The youngest patient in the series reported by ALPER (1981) was 3 years of age. KARP et al. (1974) found that 10 of their 25 (40%) patients were less than 20 years of age. However, although the true incidence in young patients remains difficult to determine (KARP et al. 1974; HENDERSON 1980; ALPER 1981) it is estimated to occur in 4%–7% of all ONSM. Childhood ONSM may differ from adult form. Unlike ONSMs in adults, there is no gender predilection. They are said to be more commonly associated with neurofibromatosis type 2. pONSMs in children often behave more aggressively, are characterized by faster growth, tend to be bilateral and show intracranial involvement in comparison to adults (LISTERNICK et al. 1997) and exhibit a more invasive growth (WALSH 1970; KARP et al. 1974; HENDERSON 1980; ALPER 1981). Moreover, bilateral cases appear to have an earlier mean age of onset of symptoms at 12.8 years (DUTTON 1992). pONSM may also occur in older individuals. Five of the patients examined by WRIGHT et al. (1980) were over 60 years of age, and one of them was a man. The oldest patient evaluated by SIBONY et al. (1984) was a 66-year-old man. The oldest patient of ALPER (1981)was 83 years old. Nevertheless, when these tumours present in middle age, the prognosis is much better (WRIGHT 1977; WRIGHT et al. 1980; CLARK et al. 1989). It has also been noted that pONSM appear at an earlier age than secondary orbital meningiomas or other intracranial meningiomas (CRAIG and GOGELA 1949; MCNAB and WRIGHT 1989). It is speculated that some or all of this age difference is presumably due to relatively smaller tumours in the orbit producing symptoms earlier than a similarly sized intracranial meningioma, especially in the region such as the sphenoid ridge.

These rare tumours have attracted a considerable amount of professional attention, including reports of ONSM being reported in association with prior radiation therapy (RT) (NEWMAN and JANE 1991). In addition, rare cases of adenocarcinoma of the lung metastatic to optic nerve sheath meningioma (ARNOLD et al. 1995) have been previously published.

Though difficult to judge conclusively from the current literature, there has been a substantial shift in treatment from surgery to "intelligent neglect" to – most recently – fractionated stereotactic radiotherapy. While a comprehensive evaluation of radiotherapy is not yet at hand, due to the benign nature of pONSM and thus decades of follow-up needed, it seems that this treatment option might in future represent the mainstay of therapy for pONSM.

Acknowledgements

Imaging kindly provided by Prof. Wibke Müller-Forell, Institute for Neuroradiology, University Hospital, Mainz.

References

Alper MG (1981) Management of primary optic nerve meningiomas. Current status – therapy in controversy. J Clin Neuroophthalmol 1:101–117

Arnold AC, Hepler RS, Badr MA, Lufkin RB, Anzai Y, Konrad PN, Vinters HV (1995) Metastasis of adenocarcinoma of the lung to optic nerve sheath meningioma. Arch Ophthalmol 113:346–351

Clark WC, Theofilos CS, Fleming JC (1989) Primary optic nerve sheath meningiomas. Report of nine cases. J Neurosurg 70:37–40

Cohn EM (1983) Optic nerve sheath meningioma: neuroradiologic findings. J Clin Neuro-Ophthalmol 3:85–89

Cooling RJ, Wright JE (1979) Arachnoid hyperplasia in optic nerve glioma: confusion with orbital meningioma. Br J Ophthalmol 63:596–599

Craig WMK, Gogela LJ (1949) Intraorbital meningiomas. Am J Ophthalmol 32:1663–1680

Cushing H, Eisenhardt L (1938) Meningiomas: their classification, regional behaviour, life history and surgical end results. Springfield, III. Charles C Thomas, pp 250–282

D'Alena PR (1964) Primary orbital meningioma. Arch Ophthalmol 71:832–836

Dandy WE (1922) Prechiasmal intracranial tumors of the optic nerves. Am J Ophthalmol 5:169–188

Dandy WE (1941) Orbital tumors: results following the transcranial operative attack. Oskar Piest, New York, pp 70–130

Dunn SN, Walsh FB (1956) Meningioma (dural endothelioma) of the optic nerve; report of a case. AMA Arch Ophthalmol 56:702–707

Dutton JJ (1992) Optic nerve sheath meningioma. Surv Ophthalmol 37:167–183

Gabibov G, Blinkov SM, Tcherekayev VA (1988) The management of optic nerve meningiomas and gliomas. J Neurosurg 68:889–893

Hart WM Jr, Burde RM, Klingele TG, Perlmutter JC (1980) Bilateral optic nerve sheath meningioma. Arch Ophthalmol 98:149–151

Henderson JW (1980) Orbital tumors, 2nd edn. Brian C. Decker, New York, pp 472–496

Hollenhorst RW Jr, Hollenhorst RW Sr, MacCarrty CS (1977) Visual prognosis of optic nerve sheath meningioma producing shunt vessels on the optic disk: the Hoyt-Spencer syndrome. Trans Am Ophthalmol Soc 75:141–163

Ingalls RG (1953) Tumors of the orbit and allied pseudo tumors: an analysis of 216 cases. Springfield III. Charles C Thomas, pp 129–148

Karp LA, Zimmerman LE, Borit A, Spencer W (1974) Primary intraorbital meningiomas. Arch Ophthalmol 91:24–28

Lindegaard J, Heegaard S, Prause JU (2002) Histopathologically verified non-vascular optic nerve lesions in Denmark 1940–1999. Acta Ophthalmol Scand 80:32–37

Listernick R, Louis DN, Packer RJ, Guttmann DH (1997) Optic pathway gliomas in children with neurofibromatosis type I: consensus statement from the NF1 Optic Glioma Task Force. Ann Neurol 41:143–149

Louis DN, Ohgaki H, Wiesler OD, Cavenee WK (2007) WHO classification of tumours of the central nervous system. IARC, Lyon

Mark LE, Kennerdell JS, Maroon JC, Rosenbaum AE, Heinz R, Johnson BL (1978) Microsurgical removal of a primary intraorbital meningioma. Am J Ophthalmol 86:704–709

Mcnab AA, Wright JE (1989) Cysts of the optic nerve three cases associated with meningioma. Eye 3:355–359

Newman SA, Jane JA (1991) Meningiomas of the optic nerve, orbit, and anterior visual pathways. In: Al-Mefty O (ed) Meningiomas. Raven Press, New York, pp 461–494

Offret G (1951) Exophthalmos. Gaz Med Fr 58:1003–1004

Probst C, Gessaga E, Leuenberger AE (1985) Primary meningioma of the optic nerve sheaths: case report. Ophthalmologica 190:83–90

Reese AB (1976) Tumors of the eye, 3rd edn. Harper and Row, New York, pp 148–153

Rootman J (1988) Diseases of the orbit. A multidisciplinary approach, JB Lippincott, London, pp 281–285

Saeed P, Rootman J, Nugent RA, White VA, Mackenzie IR, Koornneef L (2003) Optic nerve sheath meningiomas. Ophthalmology 110:2019–2030

Salazar JL, Bauer J, Frenkel M, Sugar O (1977) Bilateral optic canal meningioma. Surg Neurol 8:11–14

Samples JR, Robertson DM, Taylor JZ, Waller RR (1983) Optic nerve meningioma. Ophthalmology 90:1591–1594

Shields JA, Shields CL, Scartozzi R (2004) Survey of 1264 patients with orbital tumors and simulating lesions. The 2002 montgomery lecture, part 1. Ophthalmology 111:997–1008

Sibony PA, Krauss HR, Kennerdell JS, Maroon JC, Slamovits TL (1984) Optic nerve sheath meningioma: clinical manifestations. Ophthalmology 91:1313–1324

Spencer WH (1972) Primary neoplasms of the optic nerve and its sheaths: clinical features and current concepts of pathogenetic mechanisms. Trans Am Ophthalmol Soc 70:490–528

Trobe JD, Glaser JS, Post JD, Page LK (1978) Bilateral optic canal meningiomas: a case report. Neurosurgery 3:68–74

Vallat WM, Robin A, Bokor J, Catanzano G, De Laval M, Ronayette JP (1981) Meningioma of the optic nerve in a 2-year-old child. Apropos of a case. Bull Soc Ophtalmol Fr 81:351–353

Walsh FB (1970) Meningiomas, primary within the orbit and optic canal. In: Smith JL (ed) Neuro-Ophthalmology Symposium of the University of Miami and the Bascom Palmer Eye Institute, St. Louis, vol 5. CV Mosby, pp 240–266

Wilson WB (1981) Meningioma of the anterior visual system. Surv Ophthalmol 26:109–127

Wright JE (1977) Primary optic nerve meningiomas: clinical presentation and management. Trans Am Acad Ophthalmol Otolaryngol 83:617–625

Wright JE, Call NB, Liaricos S (1980) Primary optic nerve meningioma. Br J Ophthalmol 64:553–558

Clinical Presentation

Susanne Pitz and Helmut Wilhelm

2

CONTENTS

S. Pitz, MD, PhD
University Eye Hospital, Langenbeckstrasse 1, 55101 Mainz,
Germany

H. Wilhelm, MD, PhD
University Eye Hospital, Schleichstrasse 12–16, 72016
Tübingen, Germany

KEY POINTS

ONSM typically affects middle aged women. Ophthalmologic presentation in the vast majority of patients consists in the classical features of optic neuropathy. The vast majority of patients exhibit a variable loss of vision and/or visual field, almost always accompanied by funduscopic evidence of optic nerve pathology. Optic nerve involvement presents in one half of those affected either as a disc swelling or optic atrophy. Careful examination will virtually always reveal a reduced amplitude and velocity of pupillary light reaction, a so-called relative afferent pupillary defect. Proptosis and motility impairment may develop; however they usually are only of moderate degree. Disease progression is slow, but in many cases results in blindness if left untreated. While in the adult patient population, prognosis quo ad vitam is excellent, childhood ONSM runs a more aggressive course and may be a sign of neurofibromatosis.

Introduction

The triad of visual loss, optic nerve atrophy, and optociliary shunt vessels has for more than 30 years been regarded pathognomonic for ONSM (Dutton 1992; Frisén et al. 1973; Hollenhorst et al. 1977). However, larger case series clearly delineated that this classical presentation is only seen in one quarter to one third of patients (Carrasco and Penne 2004; Liu et al. 2003; Sibony et al. 1984). More than 90% of patients suffer from a long-standing history of a painless, progressive loss of vision and/or visual field. In his still outstanding review on ONSM, Dutton reported roughly 50% of patients presenting with a visual acuity of 20/40 or better, while one quarter had poor vision ranging at counting fingers or worse, and the remainder falling in between those two groups. A review of our patients treated by radiotherapy during the last 12 years confirm those numbers (H.Wilhelm, unpublished data). Duration of visual loss may be experienced for periods as long as 5 years prior to diagnosis. If untreated, visual impairment progresses to blindness in many cases. Surgery often accelerates visual loss due to damage to the nerves blood supply inevitable while dissecting the tumor from the nerve. There are only very few exceptions to this deceptive surgical experience. These are ONSM featuring focal tumor growth not encircling the optic nerve. Some of these exceptional cases were located rather close to the globe, but preservation of visual function has also been reported in surgical removal of a tumor confined to the optic canal (Eddleman and Liu 2007; Pitz et al. 2005; Saeed et al. 2003; Törma and Koskinen 1961).

Though the natural course of ONSM eventually leads to blindness in most of the affected eyes, prognosis quo ad vitam is excellent, and no tumor related deaths have been reported so far. However, in 5% (Dutton 1992) to 10% of cases (Turbin et al. 2002) the disease is bilateral.

ONSM arise from accumulations of meningothelial cells. Within the orbit, such accumulations of meningothelial cells are called the arachnoid villi. ONSM are regarded to arise from cap cells of these arachnoid villi. They grow within the subarachnoid space, the intact arachnoid and dura acting as a tumor "capsule". Their spread usually results in a mass encircling the optic nerve while respecting its dural sheath, exerting increasing pressure on the nerve itself as well as a progressive impairment of its vascular supply. The tumor may extend from the globe to the optic canal, and eventually exhibit continued growth into the middle cranial fossa, involve the chiasma or even the contralateral nerve. Though the pattern of growth is mainly one of growth along pre-existent anatomic pathways, invasion of the optic nerve along fibrovascular septae and vessels has been shown on a histological basis (Samples et al. 1983). Infiltration of the dura and extension into the orbital tissues is a rare event (Dutton 1992).

It is well known for intracranial meningiomas that they may arise at multiple sites simultaneously (Wilson 1981). Moreover, it has been shown during surgery that "satellite" meningiomas may not be apparent on inspection, but are proven by biopsy. It remains unclear whether such cases of "multiple" tumors should be regarded as true separate lesions, or whether they represent areas of tumor extension not demonstrable by imaging or visible during surgical procedures. Consequently, whether cases of bilateral ONSM represent two separate tumors or, as has been shown in a case by Trobe, exhibit histologically confirmed continuous growth of tumor cells along the tuberculum sellae, remains a matter of debate (Berman and Miller 2006; Trobe et al. 1978).

These growth characteristics are the basis of the clinical presentation of ONSM, consisting in a slow impairment of optic nerve function due to compromised vascular supply (venous and/or arterial), impaired axonal transport, distortion/stretching of nerve fibres, and demyelination (Carrasco and penne 2004; Dutton 1992; Miller 2004). Jaggi et al. (2007) compared CSF protein content from the optic nerve sheath in an ONSM patient (obtained during optic nerve sheath fenestration) to that obtained by lumbar puncture. Remarkably, the orbital CSF exhibited a considerably increased concentration of albumin, IgG and betra-trace protein. The authors attribute this change in protein concentration to a local compartment syndrome. This might represent another mechanism contributing to optic nerve damage in ONSM (Jaggi et al. 2007). Finally, a combination of pressure and impaired perfusion, and possibly also tumor cell infiltration, results in the classical presentation of optic neuropathy. In ONSM, this is predominantly characterized by an impairment of visual field, visual acuity and color vision.

2.2
Typical Presentation

ONSM typically affect middle aged women: while earlier studies reported 61% of affected individuals to be female, more recent investigations these found the female proportion to range higher: Sibony et al. (1984) report 68%, Turbin et al. (2002) 76.9% and two other

Table 2.1. Age at presentation

	Female	Male
Dutton (1992)	42.5 years	36.1 years
Lindegaard et al. (2002)	48.8 years	29.7 years
Turbin et al. (2002)	47.1 years	
Pitz et al. (2002)	51.5 years	

publications found that figure to range from 80 % (Pitz et al. 2002; Saeed et al. 2003), respectively. Males tend to present at a younger age: while the mean age at presentation in women is typically in their 4th to 5th decade, men present 10–15 years earlier (see Table 2.1).

There is agreement in literature that pONSM does not show a side predilection. Bilateral cases are more likely to present at younger age and strikingly often exhibit a canalicular localization: While less than 10% of unilateral ONSM are confined to the optic canal, about 40%–65% of bilateral cases represent canalicular meningiomas (Berman and Miller 2006; Dutton 1992). Bilateral ONSM is considerably more often encountered in childhood (see Sects. 2.3.1 and 2.3.2).

2.2.1
Visual Acuity

Loss of visual acuity as the presenting sign ranges at 80% in a variety of studies (Dutton 1992; Saeed et al. 2003; Sibony et al. 1984). However, a small proportion of patients presents with 20/20 or 20/15 vision. These patients nevertheless complain about a subjective loss of vision. Kupersmith et al. (1982) has pointed to the fact that investigation of contrast sensitivity might in them be more suitable to reveal the subtle impairment of visual function.

Data regarding visual acuity in ONSM patients as reported in various studies published in the last decades are remarkably similar. A recent study of 88 ONSM patients found 49% having a visual acuity of 30/50 or better, 17% having a vision of 20/60 to 20/200, 18% of less than 20/200 and 15% no light perception (Saeed et al. 2003). This parallels figures reported in Dutton's review dating from 1992, with 49% of patients featuring a visual acuity of 20/50 or better, and 15% having no light perception and Turbins data with 56.3% better than 20/40 and 8% no light perception. Among our patients, 53.9% were better than 20/40 and 15.7% had no light perception (Dutton 1992; Turbin et al. 2002; H. Wilhelm, unpublished data).

As previously mentioned, onset of visual impairment typically is longstanding (median 3 years) (Wright et al. 1989). Dutton reported a mean time interval of duration of symptoms to initial diagnosis of 42 months. One third of patients experienced symptoms for 1 year or less. Though this time interval might be shorter today in view of permanently improving imaging modalities, this underlines the slow progress of visual impairment. Egan and Lessel (2002) in a series of 16 patients observed without intervention for a mean follow-up period of 10.2 years saw four patients with stable or even slightly improved VA and fields, which emphasizes that visual loss may be exceedingly slow. Further loss of vision is gradual, resulting in a decline of one to three Snellen lines per year in the majority of patients. A small percentage of patients however may suffer from periods of rapid decline (Sibony et al. 1984).

In bilateral ONSM, loss of vision typically starts unilaterally. Impairment of vision in the fellow eye was reported to start 2–27 years later (Dutton 1992).

Saeed et al. (2003) emphasized that visual acuity at time of presentation is of prognostic value: patients presenting with a visual acuity of 20/50 or better in their study tended to retain useful vision for longer periods in comparison of those with a worse initial vision.

2.2.2
Visual Obscurations

Visual obscurations – transitory loss of vision – have been reported in 15% (Saeed et al. 2003) to 23% of patients (Sibony et al. 1984). They may to occur *prior to*, but also markedly *after*, the onset of visual loss and thus do not seem to be related to a specific stage of the disease (Sibony et al. 1984; Wright et al. 1989). They are not exclusively seen in ONSM, but are similar to those experienced by patients suffering from papilloedema due to raised intracranial pressure. Sibony and co-workers could not demonstrate any relation between occurrence of obscurations and amount of visual decline. They may occur spontaneously, posturally, or be gaze evoked (mostly on up gaze or abduction). Their duration typically is only for seconds. They may vary in frequency from a few to hundreds of episodes per day (Sibony et al. 1984; Wright et al. 1989). Wright was able to confirm the vascular etiology of this phenomenon in a patient with transient monocular blindness when abducting the eye. In fluorescein-angiography he noted a cessation of flow in the central retinal artery during abduction which turned to normal in primary position of the affected eye (Wright et al. 1989). However, *non*-gaze-dependent transient visual obscurations most presumably are not caused by a similar mechanism. Hayreh (1977) could not demonstrate any vascular abnormalities in transient visual obscurations observed in papilloedema. He postulated that obscurations occur due to a prelaminar circulatory stasis, which results in a transiently disproportionate disc perfusion in relation to the surrounding tissue pressure. Obscurations seem to subside with the development of definite optic nerve atrophy (Sibony et al. 1984).

2.2.3
Visual Field

There is no typical visual field defect in ONSM: Dutton (1992) reported one third of field defects being concentric or paracentral, respectively. While in his report an enlarged blind spot was found in 15%, Sibony et al. (1984) found this type of field defect in 32% of patients. Nerve fibre bundle defects are usually seen (Fig. 2.1a,b), but altitudinal scomtomas may be seen as well. In con-

trast, vertical hemianopic defects are very rare. Overall, there seems to be no good correlation between size and depth of field defect and loss of visual acuity.

2.2.4
Pupillary Light Response

A decreased pupillary constriction to a light stimulus on the affected side (relative afferent pupillary defect,

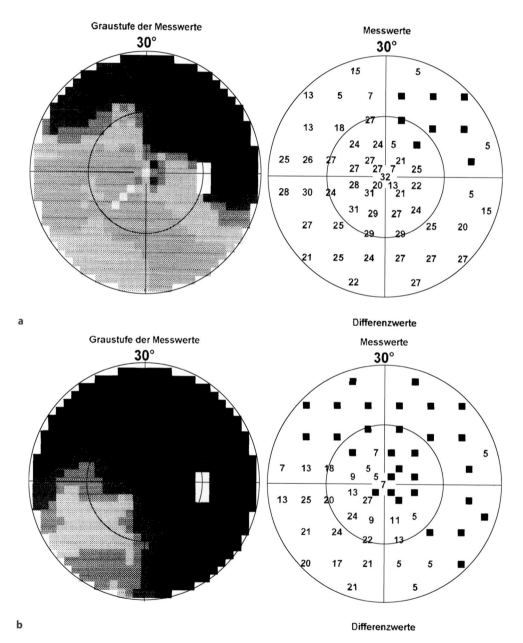

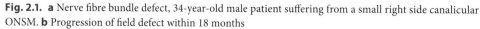

Fig. 2.1. **a** Nerve fibre bundle defect, 34-year-old male patient suffering from a small right side canalicular ONSM. **b** Progression of field defect within 18 months

RAPD) is a uniform sign of unilateral or bilateral asymmetric optic nerve affection. Sibony and co-workers report it to be present in 86% of ONSM patients, which is paralleled by our data ranging at 78.9% in our series (Sibony et al. 1984; H. Wilhelm, unpublished data). Sibony et al. report two patients without RAPD, one with one month history and a VA of 20/15, the other with a three year history of ONSM and a VA of 20/25. Both patients had normal color vision. These findings might suggest that an RAPD is missing in early phases of this disorder. However, Miller (2004) has pointed out that very subtle disturbances of pupillary reaction may missed in routine investigation. He speculated that the failure to detect an RAPD more likely is due to inadequate testing rather than to its real absence. Possibly subtle afferent defects escape clinical pupil testing, but would be detected by pupillographic techniques. We agree that RAPD is one of the earliest signs of visual impairment in ONSM and should therefore be tested carefully.

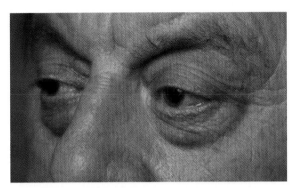

Fig. 2.2. Moderate proptosis in a 64-year-old male patient suffering from left sided ONSM

usually by about one year (Wright et al. 1989). There seems to be no correlation of proptosis and visual impairment (Saeed et al. 2003). Proptosis shows a moderate progression in a small proportion of patients (Sibony et al. 1984).

2.2.5
Color Vision

Impaired colour vision was reported to affect 73% of patients in Dutton's review. Sibony et al. (1984) only detected in 27% of their patients when testing Ishihara plates. This discrepancy is most probably due to the fact that Ishihara plates are not designed for detection of acquired, but congenital colour vision deficiencies. Impaired colour vision may not necessarily be an early sign of optic nerve dysfunction in ONSM, as it has been reported to be preceded by optic disc swelling by two years (Subramanian et al. 2004). It may be absent in single cases exhibiting optic nerve swelling and subtle visual field changes, but no RAPD. In follow-up investigations of those patients lacking an RAPD at presentation, this sign manifested within one year (Sibony et al. 1984).

2.2.6
Proptosis

The proptosis found in ONSM is usually mild with an average of 3 mm (range: 2–6 mm; Fig. 2.2). The percentage of patients reported to exhibit this sign varies from 30% to 68% in different studies (Carrasco and Penne 2004; Dutton 1992; Liu et al. 2003; Saaed et al. 2003; Sibony et al. 1984). In single cases, it may be the presenting sign of ONSM (Dutton 1992; Sibony et al. 1984). The loss of vision precedes the onset of proptosis

2.2.7
Ocular Motility

There is no characteristic pattern of misalignment or motility impairment; limitation of ductions may be found in up to 40%–50% of patients, up gaze being the most frequently limited direction (Dutton 1992; Saeed et al. 2003). Despite the high frequency of this feature, double vision seems in only experienced by about 4% of affected individuals (Saeed et al. 2003). Cranial nerve palsy is only found in 5% of ONSM patients suffering from motility impairment (Dutton 1992). Disturbance of motility seems to be more common in ONSM associated with neurofibromatosis (NF, see Sect. 2.3.2). Deterioration of motility impairment during disease progression usually is not very pronounced.

2.2.8
Anterior Segment Changes

Chemosis and lid edema may be found in rare and mostly long-standing cases (Carrasco and Penne 2004; Sibony et al. 1984).

2.2.9
Posterior Segment Changes/Optic Disc

Optic disc pathology is present in most patients, being the presenting sign in 98% (Dutton 1992). Only one

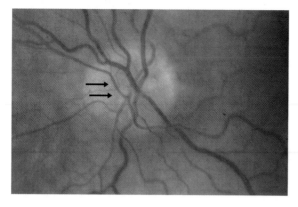

Fig. 2.3. Disc swelling with refractile bodies (*arrows*)

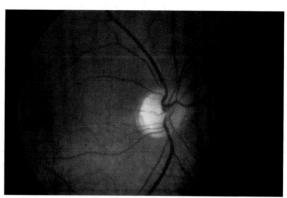

Fig. 2.4. Optic atrophy in a 34-year-old male patient suffering from right side canalicular ONSM (corresponding visual field depicted in Fig. 2.1 a,b; corresponding MRI Fig. 2.5)

out of 50 in the series of WRIGHT et al. (1989) presented with a normal disc. In our series, we saw 8% of patients with normal appearing discs (H.WILHELM, unpublished data). Disc edema (Fig. 2.3) or optic atrophy is found in about one half of the patients with pathologic findings, each (SIBONY et al. 1984, SAEED et al. 2003). As disc edema in single cases has found to be segmental it may be confused with anterior ischemic optic neuropa-

thy (AION) (GUHLMANN and KOMMERELL 1995). Disc edema seems to be less frequent in canalicular ONSM, which more frequently exhibit an atrophic disc already at initial presentation (Figs. 2.4 and 2.5). Evolution of disc edema into atrophy usually takes years. In consequence, optic atrophy is related to a more pronounced impairment of visual acuity than disc edema.

Disc edema has been reported in one third of pa-

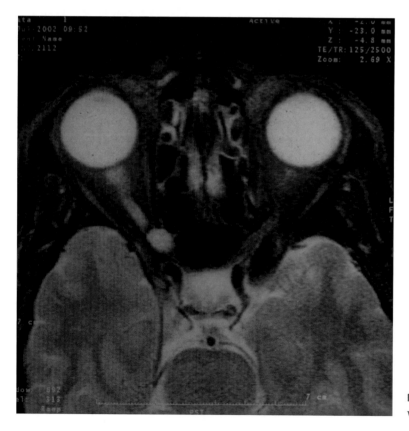

Fig. 2.5. Corresponding axial T2 weighted MRI scan

tients to be accompanied by circumpapillary retinal folds (Sibony et al. 1985). Cotton wool spots or intraretinal hemorrhage – otherwise typical findings in papilledema/raised intracranial pressure or in ischemic optic neuropathy – are rare in ONSM-related disc swelling. More chronic stages of disc edema are well known to additionally exhibit small refractile bodies on the disc (Fig. 2.3), which are smaller than the so-called drusen (hyaline bodies) of the disc. They are of yellowish colour and predominantly located in the superotemporal and inferotemporal quadrants (Sibony et al. 1985). They have been interpreted as "hard exudates" and tend to disappear with the progression of disc edema into optic atrophy. Refractile bodies are *not* specific for ONSM but have also been seen in chronic papilledema.

Venous congestion is seen as well in combination with disc edema and optic atrophy. Optociliary shunt vessels – a sign of impaired outflow through the central retinal vein leading to the opening of embryologically pre-existent retino-ciliary anastomoses – are found in one quarter to one third of affected individuals (Dutton 1992; Saeed et al. 2003; Sibony et al. 1984; Fig. 2.6). The normal route of venous outflow from the globe is through the central retinal vein in the cavernous sinus. Longstanding obstruction of the central retinal vein results in dilation of shunt vessels allowing drainage to the choroidal venous circulation, which drains as well into the superior and inferior ophthalmic veins. This retinal-choroidal flow could be confirmed by indocyanicne green angiography in ONSM patients (Muci-Mendoza et al. 1999). The time interval needed until optociliary shunt vessels appear in optic nerve compression is believed to be 1–2 years. Therefore, they are mostly encountered in cases which already developed some degree of optic atrophy. Optociliary shunt vessels are seen in other conditions than

ONSM: they may develop in other compressive optic nerve lesions, in chronic papilledema, may form after central retinal vein occlusion, and have been described in glaucoma as well as a congenital anomaly. Choroidal folds may be found in patients with higher degrees of proptosis.

2.2.10
Pain/Headache

Non-specific complaints may consist in orbital pain or headaches. Figures reporting these symptoms vary in the diverse observations, ranging from 2% to 50% (Carrasco and Penne 2004; Liu et al. 2003; Sibony et al. 1984).

2.3
Atypical Clinical Presentation

2.3.1
Childhood ONSM

Of ONSM patients, 4%–7% are younger than 20 years at onset of symptoms (Berman and Miller 2006). In contrast to the adult patient population, there is no sex predilection in pediatric ONSM patients. The youngest patient to date reported to suffer from ONSM was a 2.5-year-old female (Dutton 1992). Childhood ONSM differs from its clinical presentation in adulthood by a higher rate of intracranial extension, a higher prevalence of bilateral ONSM, and a more aggressive behavior (Dutton 1992; Eddleman and Liu 2007; Saeed et al. 2003). In Duttons meta-analysis the mean age of onset of all bilateral cases with sufficient history was 12.8 years. These differing characteristics in the pediatric patient population may at least in part be attributed to an underlying neurofibromatosis as ONSM occurs more frequently in patients suffering from neurofibromatosis (NF), especially NF 2 (see below). In Saeeds series, two out of six pediatric ONSM-patients had proven NF; two others had café au lait spots.

2.3.2
ONSM in Neurofibromatosis

The incidence of neurofibromatosis (NF) in the general population is reported to range from 0.03% to 0.05%. In contrast to these figures, Dutton's meta-analysis calculated a 9% prevalence of NF in a cohort of 142 ONSM

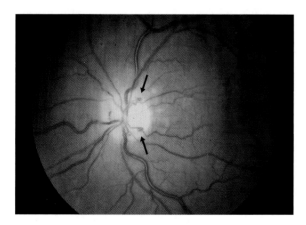

Fig. 2.6. Optociliary shunt vessels (*arrows*)

patients. Therefore, it seems reasonable to assume a more than incidental relation between NF and ONSM. Nevertheless, evidence from the current literature is incomplete, as not all studies clearly state whether NF was ruled out, or do not make a clear distinction between NF type 1 (Recklinghausen disease) and NF type 2 (central neurofibromatosis). Moreover, optic nerve glioma, which is typically found in NF 1 may exhibit considerable clinical and imaging overlap to ONSM, rendering analysis of data even more difficult.

ONSM in the context of NF presents in younger age and shows a higher rate of bilateral involvement: the mean age of adult NF patients exhibiting ONSM ranges at 35 years (Bosch et al. 2006; Cunliffe et al. 1992; Eddleman and Liu 2007; Sibony et al. 1984), which is obviously younger than the mean age of initial diagnosis of non-NF ONSM of about 41 years (Carrasco and Penne 2004; Saeed et al. 2003; Wright et al. 1989). While bilateral ONSM is reported to occur in 5%–10% of cases, bilateral involvement has been found in up to 25% of ONSM in NF type 2 (Bosch et al. 2006; Cunliffe et al. 1992; Dutton 1992). ONSM seems to be by far more frequent in NF type 2 than in NF type 1 (Wright et al. 1989). Bosch and co-workers in their study on 30 NF 2 patients found ONSM only in those 8 patients suffering from the more severe NF 2 subtype (Wishart). Visual decline, which usually is slow, was found to be more rapid in NF-related ONSM (Bosch et al. 2006). In their series five patients suffered from pONSM (one patient with bilateral involvement). Five of seven affected eyes were blind at the end of follow-up, which corresponded to a mean age of 30 years (range 14–55). Four out of these five patients exhibited marked limitations of extraocular muscle function. This study supports the view that pONSM in NF patients has a more aggressive course, leading to severely impaired visual function at a relatively early age. Optic disc appearance and visual field defects do not differ from typical ONSM cases.

2.3.3
Other Presentations

Intraocular tumor growth has been described in 3.5% of cases (Dutton 1992). Invasion most probably is via blood vessels, as meningioma cells have been demonstrated within the vascular lumina of the ciliary arteries and the central retinal vessels. Extension into the orbit after break of the tumors capsule is exceedingly rare, but may develop in longstanding cases (Carrasco and Penne 2004; Sadowski et al. 2006).

ONSM may in rare instances be the site of secondary metastasis of systemic malignancies: Arnold et al. (1995) report a histology proven case of metastasis of an adenocarcinoma of the lung to an ONSM 12 years after its initial diagnosis. While metastasis to an ONSM obviously is exceedingly rare, metastasis to the optic nerve *mimicking* ONSM is more frequent. It has up to now been reported in 11 of cases breast tumours. The clinical presentation of these metastatic cases was similar to ONSM, and in 3 out of the 11 patients there was no evidence of an underlying malignancy at inition of visual complaints (Fox et al. 2005). Survival of most of the affected patients was 4–6 months; however in one patient it was as long as 3 years.

Dabbs and Kline (1997) report a case of a 50-year-old lady suffering from repeated episodes of visual impairment and diplopia with good response to systemic steroid treatment. Imaging exhibited bilateral muscle enlargement as well as thickening of the optic nerve, enabling diagnosis of (simultaneous) Graves' orbitopathy and bilateral ONSM. This case was successfully treated by orbital irradiation. A similar case was reported by Sadowski et al. (2006).

Sometimes optic nerve sheath meningiomas may show features of an inflammation. Lessel et al. (2007) reported a case with biopsy-proven ONSM showing clinical signs recurrent orbital inflammation, improving markedly on steroids. Repeated biopsy did not show any inflammatory cells. The pathogenesis is unclear in this case however; we have seen few similar cases but did not obtain biopsy.

Ectopic orbital ONSM are reported to make up 4% of all pONSM (Dutton 1992; Rootman 2003). They are presumed to arise from ectopic arachnoid cells within the orbital connective tissue or residing along orbital nerves. The existence of such ectopic arachnoid cells is still a matter of debate, as any such have never been conclusively shown to exist (Dutton 1992). Moreover, other entities like fibroxanthomas, hemangiopericytomas and fibrous histiocytomas may be mistaken histologically for meningiomas.

Acknowledgements

Imagining kindly provided by Prof. Wibke Müller-Forell, Institute for Neuroradiology, University Hospital, Mainz.

References

Arnold AC, Hepler RS, Badr MA, Lufkin RB, Anzai Y, Konrad RN, Vinters HV (1995) Metastasis of adenocarcinoma of the lung to optic nerve sheath meningioma. Arch Ophthalmol 113:346–351

Berman D, Miller NR (2006) New concepts in the management of optic nerve sheath meningiomas. Ann Acad Med Singapore 35:168–174

Bosch MM, Wichmann WW, Boltshauser E, Landau K (2006) Optic nerve sheath meningiomas in patients with neurofibromatosis type 2. Arch Ophthalmol 124:379–385

Carrasco JR, Penne RB (2004) Optic nerve sheath meningiomas and advanced treatment options. Curr Opin Ophthalmol 15:406–410

Cunliffe IA, Moffat DA, Hary DG, Moore AT (1992) Bilateral optic nerve sheath meningiomas in a patient with neurofibromatosis type 2. Br J Ophthalmol 76:310–312

Dabbs CB, Kline LB (1997) Big muscles and big nerves. Surv Ophthalmology 42:247–254

Dutton JJ (1992) Optic nerve sheath meningiomas. Surv Ophthalmol 37:167–183

Eddelman CS, Liu JK (2007) Optic nerve sheath meningioma: current diagnosis and treatment. Neurosurg Focus 23:E5

Egan RA, Lessel S (2002) A contribution to the natural history of optic nerve sheath meningiomas. Arch Ophthalmol 120:1505–1508

Fox B, Pacheco P, DeMonte F (2005) Carcinoma of the breast metastatic to the optic nerve mimicking an optic nerve sheath meningioma: case report and review of the literature. Skull Base 15:281–287

Frisén L, Hoyt WF, Tengroth BM (1973) Optociliary veins, disc pallor and visual loss: a triad of signs indicating spheno-orbital meningioma. Acta Ophthalmol (Copenh) 51:241–249

Guhlmann M, Kommerell G (1995) Simulation of anterior ischemic optic neuropathy by optic nerve sheath meningioma. Klin Monatsbl Augenheilk 207:200–202

Hayreh SS (1977) Optic disc edema in raised intracranial pressure. Arch Ophthalmol 95:1566–1579

Hollenhorst RW Jr, Hollenhorst RW Sr, MacCarty CS (1977) Visual prognosis of optic nerve sheath meningiomas producing shunt vessels on the optic disc: the Hoyt-Spencer syndrome Trans Am Ophthalmol Soc 75:141–163

Jaggi GP, Mironow A, Huber AR, Killer HE (2007) Optic nerve compartment syndrome in a patient with optic nerve sheath meningioma. Eur J Ophthalmol 17:454–458

Kupersmith MJ, Siegel IM, Carr RE (1982) Subtle disturbances of vision with compressive lesions of the anterior visual pathway measured by contrast sensitivity. Ophthalmology 89:68–72

Lessell S, Kim JW, Hatton MP, Stemmer-Rachamimov A, Thiagalingham S, Rubin PA (2007) Clinical without histopathological manifestations of inflammation in a patient with primary intraorbital optic nerve sheath meningioma. J Neuroophthalmol 27:104–106

Lindegaard J, Heegaard S, Prause JU (2002) Histopathologically verified non-vascular optic nerve lesions in Denmark 1940-99. Acta Ophthalmol Scand 80:32–37

Liu JK, Forman S, Moorthy CR, Benzil DL (2003) Update on treatment modalities for optic nerve sheath meningiomas. Neurosurg Focus 14:E7

Miller NR (2004) Primary tumours of the optic nerve and its sheaths. Eye 18:1026–1037

Muci-Mendoza R, Arevalo JF, Ramella M, Fuenmayor-Rivera D, Karam E, Cardenas PL, Recio MV (1999) Optociliary veins in optic nerve sheath meningioma. Indocyanine green videoangiographic findings. Ophthalmology 106:311–318

Pitz S, Becker G, Schiefer U, Wilhelm H, Jeremic B, Bamberg M, Zrenner E (2002) Stereotactic fractionated irradiation of optic nerve sheath meningioma: a new treatment alternative. Br J Ophthalmol 86:1265–1268

Pitz S, Schwenn O, Bittinger F, Müller-Forell WS (2005) Successful surgical treatment of a primary optic nerve sheath meningioma. Neuro-Ophthalmology 29:121–123

Rootman J (2003) Diseases of the orbit. A multidisciplinary approach. JB Lippincott, London pp 233–240

Sadowki B, Wöhrle R, Wörhle N, Helmke K (2006) Protrusio bulbi. Ophthalmologe 103:810–814

Saeed P, Rootman J, Nugent RA, White VA, Mackenzie IR, Korneef L (2003) Optic nerve sheath meningiomas. Ophthalmology 110:2019–2030

Samples JR, Robertson DM, Taylor JZ, Waller RR (1983) Optic nerve sheath meningioma. Ophthalmology 90:1591–1594

Sibony PA, Krauss HR, Kennerdell JS, Maroon JC, Slamovits TL (1984) Optic nerve sheath meningiomas. Clinical manifestations. Ophthalmology 91:1313–1324; discussion by Miller NR. Ophthalmology 91:1324–1326

Sibony PA, Kennerdell JS, Slamovits TL, Lessel S, Krauss HR (1985) Intrapapillary refractile bodies in optic nerve sheath meninigioma. Arch Ophthalmol 103:383–385

Subramanian PS, Bressler NM, Miller NR (2004) Radiation retinopathy after fractionated stereotactic radiotherapy for optic nerve sheath meningioma. Ophthalmology 111:565–567

Törma T, Koskinen K (1961) A case of unilateral optic foramen meningioma. Acta Ophthalmol 39:460–465

Trobe JD, Glaser JS, Post JD, Page LK (1978) Bilateral optic canal meningiomas: a case report. Neurosurgery 3:68–74

Turbin RE, Thompson CR, Kennerdell JS, Cockerham KP, Kupersmith MJ (2002) A long-term visual outcome comparison in patients with optic nerve sheath meningioma managed with observation, surgery, radiotherapy, or surgery and radiotherapy. Ophthalmology 109:890–899; discussion 899-900; comment in Ophthalmology (2002)109:833–834; Ophthalmology (2003) 110:1282–1283; author reply 1283

Wilson WB (1981) Meningiomas of the anterior visual system. Surv Ophthalmol 26:109–125

Wright JE, McNab AA, McDonald WI (1989) Primary optic nerve sheath meningioma. Br J Ophthalmol 73:960–966

3

Clinical Evaluation of Primary Optic Nerve Sheath Meningioma

Roger E. Turbin and John S. Kennerdell

CONTENTS

KEY POINTS

Optic nerve sheath meningioma (ONSM) may develop anywhere along the course of the optic nerve, from globe to prechiasmal, intracisternal optic nerve. As progressive visual loss occurs, clinical abnormalities become more developed, making the diagnosis of a compressive lesion more straightforward. As tumor extension develops within the extradural, subdural and subarachnoid space at the orbital, canalicular, or intracranial nerve segments, neuro-imaging abnormalities become more apparent. Clinical evaluation should be directed toward early identification of progressive disease. Direct invasion into surrounding orbital structures is infrequent, although intracranial spread, progressive chiasmal or contralateral optic nerve involvement, and post-operative recurrence are all documented. Although most meningioma are histologically benign and have slow progression, aggressive behavior is seen on occasion and may mimic other neoplasia or inflammatory conditions. Until recently, controlled long-term comparisons of various treatment techniques had been unavailable, adding to the controversy in managing these unusual tumors.

R.E. Turbin, MD, FACS
Assistant Professor, Neuro-ophthalmology and Orbital Surgery, University of Medicine and Dentistry-New Jersey Medical School (UMDNJ-NJMS), 90 Bergen Street, Suite 6177, Newark, NJ 07103, USA

J.S. Kennerdell, MD
Chairman and Professor Emeritus, Allegheny General Hospital, 320 East North Ave, Suite 116, Pittsburgh, PA 15212, USA

3.1
Introduction

Primary optic nerve sheath meningioma (ONSM) in most cases is a slow growing benign tumor that causes progressive ipsilateral, unilateral loss of vision, and occasionally ocular motility disorder, proptosis, or orbital congestion. However, both rapid clinical progression as well as inexorably slow clinical progression each contribute to confusion and failure to diagnose this entity accurately. Because the affected structures are typically isolated to the anterior visual pathways, the individual is free of neurologic or systemic signs and symptoms to suggest the presence of a tumor, except in the context of syndromes such as neurofibromatosis II. Therefore, few patients suffer other disease related morbidity or mortality, except in the cases of treatments gone awry, with complication rate dependant on treatment modality (13%–66.7%) (BECKER et al. 2002; TURBIN and POKORNY 2004). This chapter will discuss the clinical evaluation of primary ONSM in the context of pathophysiologic mechanism of disease.

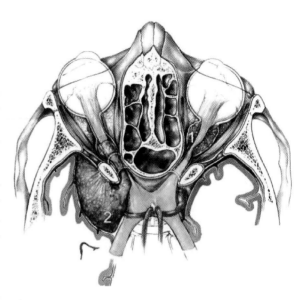

Fig. 3.1. Illustration is an artist´s representation of (1) primary intraorbital perioptic and (2) secondary optic nerve sheath meningioma. Secondary meningiomas that affect the optic nerve and orbit arise from the sphenoid ridge (inner, medial, or outer portions), suprasellar area (tuberculum sellae and parasellar), cavernous sinus, olfactory groove, intracanalicular and intraorbital optic nerve. From Bosch MM, Wichmann WW, Boltshauser E, Landau K (2006) Optic nerve sheath meningiomas in patients with neurofibromatosis type 2. Arch Ophthalmol 124(3):379–385

3.2
Meningioma of the Optic Nerve and Orbit

Primary and secondary meningiomas that affect the optic nerve and orbit arise from the sphenoid ridge (inner, medial, or outer portions), suprasellar area (tuberculum sellae and parasellar), cavernous sinus, olfactory groove, intracanalicular and intraorbital optic nerve (Fig. 3.1). These lesions invade the optic canal and orbit by extending via intradural or extradural paths from their site of origin. Approximately 90% of meningiomas that invade the orbit derive from secondary, extraorbital intracranial locations. Presenting orbital and visual signs and symptoms reflect location, extent, and duration of involvement of visual apparatus and orbital/adenexal structures. However, short of contrasting the presentation of primary and secondary forms of meningioma that affect the optic nerve, the discussion in this chapter will be limited to primary optic nerve sheath meningiomas (ONSM) (intraorbital optic nerve, canalicular optic nerve, and intracranial optic nerve).

The other forms of meningioma that affect the visual pathways and orbit typically do so secondarily from spread from adjacent structures. Appropriate evaluation therefore requires detailed clinical examination and neuro-imaging of the structures of the skull base and cavernous sinus, with special attention to the function of each of the cranial nerves. Although sharing some similarities in presentation, intrinsic differences in the ultra structural anatomy also lend secondary optic nerve meningiomas to be more amendable to surgical intervention, although divided dose conformal, hypofractionated radiotherapy and stereotactic radiosurgical methods are efficacious (RINGEL et al. 2007; SCHICK and HASSLER 2005; CRISTANTE 1994; KONDZIOLKA et al. 2008; MATHIESON and KIHLSTRÖM 2006; PEELE et al. 1996). Conversely, the surgical management of primary ONSM has limited indications and will be discussed in a subsequent chapter (TURBIN et al. 2002, 2006).

3.2.1
Primary Optic Nerve Sheath Meningioma Defined

Primary ONSM may originate from the orbit, the intracanalicular optic nerve, or the intracranial optic nerve) (near the intracranial dural falciform ligament at the base of the optic canal). The latter two forms are occa-

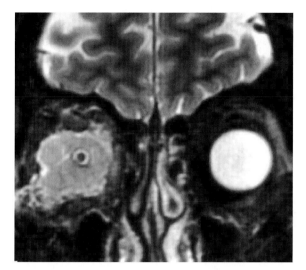

Fig. 3.2. T2 coronal weighted MRI of a subsequently biopsy proven (resection) right ONSM with penetration through dural sheath and invasion of surrounding orbital structures. The image shows irregular tumor surface with invasion into surrounding orbital fat. In this section, the optic nerve configuration with surrounding rim of high T2 weighted CSF signal appears preserved. Courtesy of Steve Newman, MD

sionally difficult to differentiate from secondary meningioma originating from adjacent structures. Synonymously known as perioptic meningioma, ONSM tend to spread along paths of least resistance, and may course along the optic nerve in subarachnoid space, invade optic nerve at pial septa as well as piercing vessels, or invade the dura and spread into adjacent orbital tissues (Fig. 3.2) (Probst et al. 1985; Mehra et al. 1979; Karp et al. 1974). Rarely the tumor may invade ocular structures such as the choroid, sclera, or optic disc (Dutton 1992; Karp et al. 1974; Schittkowski et al. 1999; Amoli et al. 2007; Coston 1936).

3.2.2
Disease Specific Limitation of Retrospective Review

Primary ONSM grow in different patterns, present at different levels of severity, and affect different regions of the optic nerve. In my opinion, the historical stratification and classification of statistical distributions of signs and symptoms have limited applicability, partially related to changing trends and advances in early detection of these lesions. It is therefore difficult to draw

modern conclusions from metanalysis of historical data designed to "review of as much of the published literature as possible" which often spanned the era prior to modern imaging (Dutton 1992). Furthermore, data are necessarily plagued by biases of reporting, data acquisition, and dissimilar evaluators, all of which are common to retrospective multicenter studies. In addition, meta-analyses from multiple centers may be based at least partially on the same patient population, and study results should be carefully considered concerning this factor (Turbin and Pokorny 2004).

In reviewing the literature, another difficulty arises related to the diagnosis of primary ONSM, which is frequently based on radiographic criteria without histopathologic confirmation. Therefore, cases defined as ONSM and treated as such by the literature are only presumed and some could represent different disease entities. However, this approach to diagnosis is consistent with our current standard of care (Turbin et al. 2002). It is clear that our improved ability to diagnose early and accurately is related to tremendous advancements in modern CT and MRI techniques. Therefore the metanalysis, combined with a few of the larger studies published since Dutton's report of 477 ONSM, continue to represent the best epidemiologic data that we have on this rare disease, acknowledging that retrospective analysis clearly may introduce bias (Dutton 1992; Saeed et al. 2003; Turbin et al. 2002; Egan and Lessell 2002; Andrews et al. 2002).

3.3
Epidemiology

ONSM are uncommon tumors accounting for 1%–2% of all meningiomas, but the estimate of incidence varies by case series, practice referral pattern, and availability of modern computed tomography (CT) and contrasted magnetic resonance imaging (MRI) with fat suppression technique (Miller 2006). For instance, Cushing and Eisenhardt (1938) described only a single meningioma arising from the optic nerve sheath in his series of 313 meningiomas. Modern estimates suggest approximately one third of optic nerve tumors are meningioma. From Dutton's literature summary, patients presented between 2.5 and 78 years of age, and only 4% of patients were less than 20 years of age. There was female predominance, but men presented at a slightly younger age (36.1 years vs 42.5). Most cases (92%) of primary ONSM originated from the intraorbital segment, and only approximately 5% were bilateral at initial presentation (Table 3.1).

Table 3.1. Epidemiologic characteristics and location of optic sheath meningiomas

Age (256)	Mean	Range
Females	42.5 years	2.5–73 years
Males	36.1 years	10–78 years
All patients	40.8 years	2.5–78 years
Sex (356)	Female 217 (61%)	Male 139 (39%)
Laterality	Unilateral 475 (95%)	Bilateral 23 (5%)
Sites of origin for meningioma involving the orbit (5000 cases)		
Secondary tumors, intracranial origin		4502 (90%)
Primary tumors, orbital origin		498 (10%)
Optic Sheath		477 (96%)
Orbital optic nerve		438 (92%)
Optic canal		40 (8%)
Ectopic		21 (4%)

Adapted from Table 1 in Dutton JJ (1992) Optic nerve sheath meningiomas. Surv Ophthalmol 37(3):167–183

3.3.1
Clinical Signs and Symptoms

Commonly reported clinical manifestations of ONSM include ipsilateral visual loss, afferent pupillary defect, color vision disturbance, visual field defect, proptosis, optic disc edema, ocular motility disturbance, and eyelid edema (especially lower eyelid). Patients have symptoms of gradual or rapid visual loss, diplopia, pain, transient visual obscuration prior to visual loss, or gaze-evoked obscurations (especially apical tumors) (TURBIN and POKORNY 2004). Initial or subsequent ophthalmoscopic examination may reveal optic nerve head swelling, contiguous macular edema (Fig. 3.3), nerve pallor, retinal, or choroidal folds. Authors have suggested choroidal folds are directly related to mass effect of anterior tumors on the globe, but we have seen choroidal folds in a patient with temporal pallor and a biopsy proven ipsilateral ONSM at the posterior entrance of the optic canal. Optic disc swelling, accompanied by optic nerve pallor, also may be observed. The reader is directed to Sects. 2.1.1–2.1.10 in Chap. 2 for additional detail. The typically mild proptosis produced by this space occupying lesion has been attributed by some authors

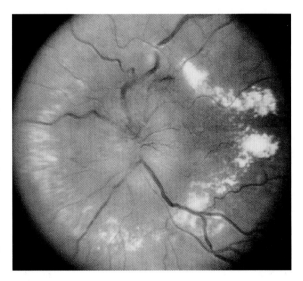

Fig. 3.3. Severe left optic nerve head edema with contiguous exudative macular edema in a patient with biopsy proven ONSM. The optic nerve head and macular edema resolved after nerve sheath biopsy. From Turbin RE, Wladis EJ, Frohman LP et al. (2006) Role for surgery as adjuvant therapy in optic nerve sheath meningioma. Ophthal Plast Reconstr Surg 22(4):278–282

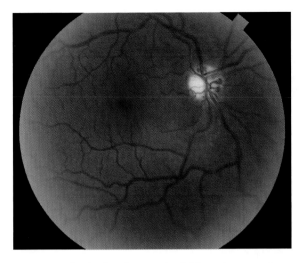

Fig. 3.4. Color fundus photograph of right optic nerve, showing prominent right optic nerve head shunt vessels in a patient with ONSM and pale optic atrophy. Courtesy of Steve Newman, MD

to represent "straightening" of the nerve sheath in addition to pure mass effect within the orbit. The careful examiner will include both exophthalmometry as well as the determination of the presence of resistance to digital retropulsion of the globe.

Growth occurs, although it may not be detected on neuroimaging studies as visual function declines. With passage of time, the optic disc edema may resolve, leaving a pale optic nerve head subject to progressive visual loss. Optociliary shunts only occasionally develop, representing secondary dilation of retinal-to choroidal shunting veins (Fig. 3.4). Progressive optic atrophy may be difficult to detect without vigilant attention to serial visual acuity, visual field, and nerve fiber layer loss. It is common in my practice to identify ONSM in patients whose progressive complaints indeed correlate to undetected decline in visual function, not detected by an unwary clinician. Careful serial photography and serial assessment of nerve fiber layer thickness are increasingly available and may identify progressive visual dysfunction in patients thought to have etiogies related to other non-neoplastic optic nerve disease.

Dutton found the most common presenting symptom to be loss of visual acuity, followed by abnormal color vision and visual fields. The incidence of visual acuity loss, blindness, optic atrophy, disc swelling, and proptosis varies somewhat by series, referral pattern of the examining physician, and radiographic historical

era at presentation. The lower overall differences in the distribution of patients with proptosis, optic disc edema, and motility disorder in the Turbin (37.7%, 43.1%, 30.2) vs Rootman series (59%, 48%, 47%) spanning a similar time frame may represent referral bias of access to tertiary healthcare. In addition, 56.3% of patients presented with visual acuity between 20/20 and 20/40 in the Turbin series compare to Dutton's 45%. This may represent the trend towards earlier diagnosis in later years. Data presented by the Turbin series is truncated because only patients with at least 50 months of follow-up were included in the series (DUTTON 1992; SAEED et al. 2003; ROOTMAN 2003; TURBIN and POKORNY 2004). The signs and symptoms are provided below from Dutton's (1887–1991), Rootman's (1976–1999) and Turbin's (1976–1999) series (Tables 3.2–3.5).

3.3.2
Characteristics of Optic Atrophy

The classic article by TROBE et al. (1980) identified the difficulty that even experienced observers have in distinguishing optic atrophy of compressive lesions from other causes. In a classic study, five experienced ophthalmologists reviewed fundus stereophotographs. Although certain features were helpful in identifying noncompressive lesions, the optic atrophy resulting from optic neuritis, compressive, traumatic, and hereditary optic neuropathies were distinguished successfully less than 50%. Useful distinguishing fundoscopic features included retinal arterial narrowing and sheathing in ischemic CRAO or ION; superior or inferior sectoral disc pallor was suggestive in ION, and temporal pallor with selective loss of central visual field in toxic optic neuropathy and optic neuritis.

The optic atrophy resulting from ONSM most often is not reliably distinguished by fundoscopic examination only. However, there may occasionally be hints in some cases. Specifically, the triad of vision loss, optic atrophy and optociliary shunt veins has been described by authors to be strongly associated with ONSM (FRISEN et al. 1973; SALZMANN 1893; ELSCHNIG 1898). The triad has however been described with glioma, sphenoid wing meningioma, chronic atrophic papilledema, CRVO and glaucoma (FRISEN et al. 1973; JAKOBIEC et al. 1984). The evolution of collateral channels shunting blood from the central retinal vein to peripapillary choroid by dilation of preformed capillary vessels following resolution of disc edema caused by ONSM is well documented in the literature (IMES et al. 1985). Frisen and colleagues argued the shunt vessels were probably preceded by long-standing edema.

Table 3.2. Clinical signs and symptoms of ONSM from Dutton's meta analysis of the literature through 1992

Condition	No. pts. with data available	No pts. Affected (%)
Decreased vision[a]	380	365(96)
Decreased visual field		112(83)
Peripheral constriction		39(35)
Central,ceco-central,paracetral		32(29)
Altitudinal		18(16)
Enlarged blind spot		15(13)
Decreased color vision	45	33(73)
Proptosis	241	142(59)
Disc atrophy	177	87(49)
Disc swelling	208	100(48)
Decreased motility	258	121(47)
Optociliary shunts	238	71(30)

[a]20/20–20/40 (45%); 20/50–20/400 (31%); CF-NLP (24%)
Adapted from Table 2 in Dutton JJ (1992) Optic nerve sheath meningiomas. Surv Ophthalmol 37(3):167–183

Table 3.3. Presenting signs and symptoms of ONSM from a single author's experience representing a referral practice from the University of British Columbia

Clinical Presentation	% of Series
Decreased vision	80
Transient visual obscurations	15
Pain	7
Diplopia	4
SIGNS	
Optic disc atrophy	55
Optic disc swelling	42
Extraocular muscle deviation or restriction	39
Proptosis	30
Optociliary shunts	25

From Table 9-5, Rootman (2003) Diseases of the orbit. A multidisciplinary approach, 2nd edn. Lipincott Williams & Wilkins, Philadelphia, page 233

Table 3.4. Clinical characteristics at presentation in 64 patients with ONSM

Descriptor	Present	Absent	Unknown
Right eye	30 (51.7%)	(excluding bilateral disease)	
Left eye	28 (48.3%)	(excluding bilateral disease)	
Both eyes	6 (9.4%)		
Proptosis	23 (37.7%)	38	3
Nerve head edema	22 (43.1 %)	29	13
APD	56 (93.3%)	4	4
Motility abnormality	19 (30.2%)	44	1
Shunt vessels	4*	(Likely underreported)	

*One additional patient developed shunt vessels one year after diagnosis. APD = afferent pupillary defect.

From Table 3, Turbin RE, Thompson CR, Kennerdell JS, Cockerham KP, Kupersmith MJ (2002) A long-term visual outcome comparison in patients with optic nerve sheath meningioma managed with observation, surgery, radiotherapy, or surgery and radiotherapy. Ophthalmology 109(5):890–899

Table 3.5. Initial and final visual data in 64 patients with primary ONSM

	1.0 to 0.5	0.4 to 0.05	Less than 0.05			
Initial visual acuity (ratio)	36 (56.3%)	8 (12.5%)	20 (31.3%)			
Final visual acuity (ratio)	18 (28.1%)	10 (15.6%)	36 (56.3%)			
	0	1	>0.3	<0.3		Unknown
Initial color vision*	29 (51.8%)	10 (17.9%)	20 (35.7%)	36 (64.3%)		8
Final color vision*	42 (77.8%)	6 (11.1%)	10 (18.5%)	44 (81.5%)		10
	0	1	2	3	4	Unknown
Initial field grade†	6 (9.7%)	20 (32.3%)	10 (16.1%)	20 (32.3%)	6 (9.7%)	2
Final field grade†	5 (8.1 %)	8 (12.9%)	10 (16.1%)	13 (21.0%)	26 (41.9%)	2

*Color vision presented as decimal ratio of number of correct Ishihara color plates divided by total number of plates tested, excluding control plate. 0 = no plate correct, 0.5 = one half of color plates tested correctly. Percentages are calculated of known values after excluding unknown values from the denominator.

†Visual field grading scale; 0 = normal field; 1 = arcuate field deficit or mild general depression; 2 = relative central (less than 6 degrees), or cecocentral, or altitudinal; 3 = altitudinal plus additional loss or very severe constriction; 4 = no light perception.

From Table 2, Turbin RE, Thompson CR, Kennerdell JS, Cockerham KP, Kupersmith MJ (2002) A long-term visual outcome comparison in patients with optic neve sheath meningioma managed with observation, surgery, radiotherapy, or surgery and radiotherapy. Ophthalmology 109(5):890–899

3.3.3
Growth Patterns

In general terms, primary ONSM progression is associated with chronic optic nerve compression and occasionally invasion of the nerve as in other forms of meningioma that involve cranial nerves (LARSON et al. 1995; SEN and HAGUE 1997). This causes typically painless, progressive loss of visual function, and signs of optic neuropathy including ipsilateral relative afferent pupillary defect, optic atrophy and nerve fiber layer loss that may be preceded by optic nerve head swelling. Patients may experience other symptoms and signs detailed above (Tables 3.2–3.5), and the pattern of involvement is typically reflected by extent, severity and duration of disease, as in other forms of compressive optic neuropathies. It is therefore germane to introduce some detail concerning growth patterns and pathophysiology which will be discussed in subsequent chapters.

3.3.3.1
Growth Patterns Defined

The classification of general growth patterns has been detailed over the years by various authors, but Rootman's classification of four patterns (tubular, globular, fusiform, or focal) is a clinically relevant summary of tumor configuration (Figs. 3.5–3.9). He further subdivided the tubular pattern into tubular-diffuse, tubular with apical, and tubular with anterior expansion (Table 3.6). The combined experience (88 patients) of the University of British Columbia series and the University of Amsterdam between 1976 and 1999 (SAEED et al. 2003) was described in both Rootman's textbook and a recent retrospective study (ROOTMAN 2003; SAEED et al. 2003). However, with the exception of the tubular pattern with apical expansion which demonstrated the worst visual prognosis, no correlation was found between ONSM configuration and visual outcome in his series. The authors do cite the trend towards early visual loss, and a higher tendency toward intracranial extension in patients with intracanalicular ONSM. Of all patients, 27% suffered no light perception vision (NLP) before intervention. Calcified lesions increased in volume by 3.38 mm^3 and in length by 0.12 mm per year, and non-calcified lesions grew six times faster, increasing in volume by 23.45 mm^3 and in length by 0.6 mm per year (ROOTMAN 2003; SAEED et al. 2003).

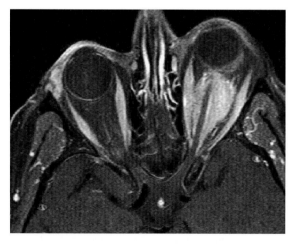

Fig. 3.5. T1 weight MRI with contrast enhanced, fat suppression technique reveals a globular left ONSM. Tumor is represented by enhancing mass extending from left globe to orbital apex, with slight early enhancement extending into left optic canal. *Courtesy of Roger Turbin, MD

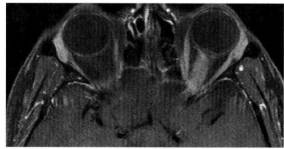

Fig. 3.6. T1 weight MRI with contrast enhanced fat suppression technique reveals a tubular left ONSM extending from left globe up, through left optic canal, to the intracranial optic nerve. Courtesy of Roger Turbin, MD

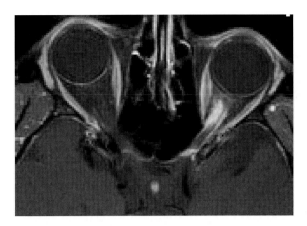

Fig. 3.7. T1 fat suppressed gadolinium enhanced example of another tubular left ONSM with intraorbital, intracanalicular (tramtracking), and intracranial optic nerve involvement. Note the appearance of a thin line of contrast enhancement, or "tram-track" through the optic canal. In cases of isolated intracanalicular meningioma, this subtle sign is easily overlooked. Courtesy of Roger Turbin, MD

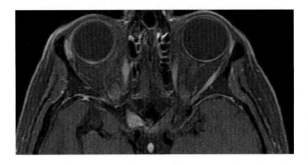

Fig. 3.8. Focal meningioma affecting the right intracranial optic nerve segment, shown with T1 fat suppressed axial MRI. Courtesy of Roger Turbin, MD

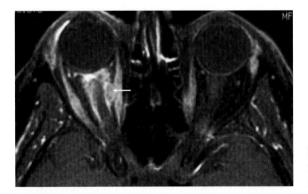

Fig. 3.9. A predominantly focal right ONSM, shown on contrast enhanced T1 axial image with fat suppression. Courtesy of Steve Newman, MD

Table 3.6. Configuration of optic nerve sheath meningiomas as seen on imaging (n = 74 optic nerves)

Configuration	Number	Optic Cancal Involvement	Intracranial Involvement	Tram Tracking	Clacification		Irregular Margins
					Dense	Scatter	
Tubular							
Diffuse	33	20	11	11	11	3	3
Apical expansion	11	8	7	4	3	0	1
Anterior expansion	2	0	0	0	0	0	0
Globular	17	6	2	3	3	1	9
Fusiform	8	3	1	1	1	0	2
Focal enlargement of optic nerve	3	0	0	0	0	1	0
Total	74	37	21	19	18	5	15

From Saeed P, Rootman J, Nugent RA et al. (2003) Optic nerve sheath meningiomas. Ophthalmology 110(10):2019–2030

3.3.3.2
Variations in Growth Pattern and Location Affect Symptoms

Variation in growth pattern may cause vision to be affected at different rates and different stage of disease. Numerous authors have quoted Clark's description that anterior nerve sheath meningioma located behind the globe may spread extradurally or in a more relaxed fashion in the area where the nerve sheath inserts onto the posterior globe, limiting compression of the nerve and preserving vision until late in the course. With increased growth, these patients may present with proptosis prior to visual loss (Figs. 3.10 and 3.11). Some tumors, before they spread to reach the distal optic nerve, cause a cystic expansion of the distal perioptic optic space (LINDBLOM et al. 1992a, b; MCNABB and WRIGHT 1989; FRASIER and GREEN 2002) or a cystic expansion of the meningioma itself (Figs. 3.12 and 3.13) (LAITT et al. 1996; BOSCH et al. 2006).

Posterior tumors may be more confined to the dura and expand within the sheath, causing chronic compression or actual optic nerve invasion, which contributes to choking off of the blood supply and limitation of axoplasmic flow. These changes lead to loss of vision and optic atrophy, often with only limited proptosis. This may occur with or without preceding optic disc swelling (CLARK et al. 1989). A similar presentation with

earlier visual loss and optic atrophy has been described with intracanalicular ONSM, a location which provides little room for growth before atrophy sets in (ORTIZ et al. 1996; CASTEL et al. 2000; JACKSON 2003). However, cases of posterior involvement with swelling of the optic nerve do occur (LINDBLOM 1992b). Although intracanalicular and posterior orbital lesions may rarely be associated with disc swelling (KENNERDELL and MAROON 1975), almost all cases with disc swelling affect the more anterior orbit (LINDBLOM 1992b),

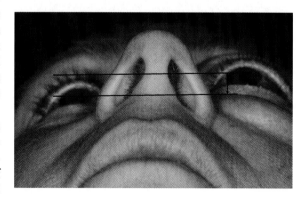

Fig. 3.10. Clinical photograph of 8 mm of left proptosis in a patient with a left anterior, intraorbital ONSM and 20/20 vision OU. Courtesy of Roger Turbin, MD

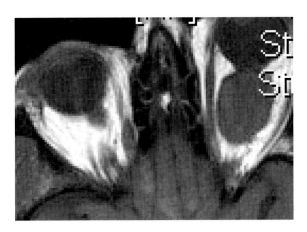

Fig. 3.11. The relatively anterior left intraorbital ONSM presumably allowed for peripheral expansion with little actual optic nerve compression, preserving visual acuity with 15 years of follow-up, in the same patient shown in Fig. 3.10. Courtesy of Roger Turbin, MD

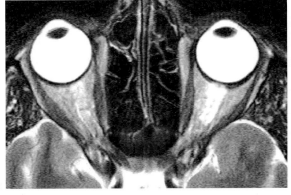
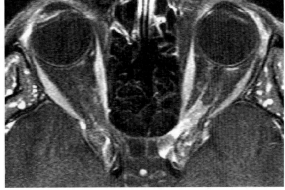

a

b

Fig. 3.12. a Cystic expansion of the left perioptic space in a patient with a predominantly intracanalicular ONSM with extension into the orbital apex. This is demonstrated as bright signal on this T2 weighted axial image. **b** The T1 fat sup-pressed image demonstrates predominantly intracanalicular ONSM with tubular extension into the left orbital apex, shown as plaque like enhancement in the same patient. Courtesy of Roger Turbin, MD

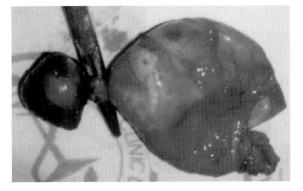

Fig. 3.13. Gross pathology of resected massive cystic expansion of optic nerve meningioma. Cystic change is more common in optic nerve glioma. From Rosca TI, Carstocea BD, Vlădescu TG (2006) Cystic optic nerve sheath meningioma. J Neuroophthalmol 26(2):121–122

Special Cases

Specific forms of ONSM present unique characteristics and diagnostic challenges related to clinical characteristics. These subtypes of ONSM are presented below.

3.4.1
The Intracanalicular Meningioma

Susac, Smith and Walsh originally coined the term "impossible meningioma" to refer to virtually undetectable apical ONSM prior to modern techniques of neuroimaging, but the intracanalicular ONSM most strongly exemplifies the concept given our persistent difficulty in establishing the radiographic diagnosis and distinguishing the lesion from other diseases (ALPER and SHERMAN 1989; SUSAC et al. 1977). Optic canal meningiomas may present early with visual loss, or optic atrophy without swelling due to posterior location and inability of the nerve to tolerate small degrees of compression within the optic canal. Optic neuropathy associated with enlargement of posterior aerated ethmoid and sphenoid sinus is termed pneumosinus dilitans, and may represent a clue to an adjacent intracanalicular meningioma (HIRST et al. 1979; MILLER et al. 1996). The intracanalicular meningioma location also has the highest incidence of bilaterality (DUTTON 1992).

JACKSON et al. (2003) recently summarized their experience with six cases, each with delay of diagnosis for greater than 1 year after onset of symptoms. Each occurred in a young woman between the ages of 24 and 38 years, 4 with rapid initial onset (one painful) and the remaining 2 with rapid progression of symptoms weeks after repeated episodes of transient visual loss. In each case a diagnosis of optic neuritis was made and the correct diagnosis of intracanalicular ONSM was not confirmed until the patient suffered progressive visual loss after intravenous corticosteroid therapy. The radiographic characteristics that contrast the intracanalicular meningioma from other disease processes will be described subsequently in later chapters. However, fat suppressed MRI with contrast may define thin "tram-tracking" of enhancement within the optic canal that may be the only radiographic sign of an intracanalicular ONSM (Fig. 3.7). In other cases, CT may demonstrate a line of calcification within the tumor, or perioptic hyperostosis in the surrounding optic canal.

3.4.2
Meningioma in Neurofibromatosis

Patients with NF 1 and NF 2, which occur in the general population at 0.04% and 0.0025%, respectively, have been cited to a harbor a higher incidence of both intracranial meningioma and ONSM (EVANS et al. 2005; CREANGE et al. 1999). However, the two entities have been confused in the literature until the relatively recent molecular delineation of NF 1 and 2 at two different chromosomal loci. Landau and colleagues performed a literature review and added their cumulative experience of patients with ONSM (1991–2003) and found an overall incidence of meningioma in NF 2 of 6.8% (BOSCH et al. 2006). Interestingly, the experience (27%) of their institution included 8 cases of meningioma in 30 patients with NF2. Furthermore, the authors reanalyzed 16 cases of ONSM associated with neurofibromatosis from the literature, and concluded that 10 had NF2, and 6 lacked enough clinical information to differentiate neurofibromatosis subtype (ALS 1969; CUNLIFFE et al. 1992; CIBIS et al. 1985; SWENSON et al. 1982; PARKER 1922; HARTMANN 1933; SHAPLAND and GREENFIELD 1935; WORSTER et al. 1937; WALSH 1970; KARP et al. 1974; JACOBIEC et al. 1984; WRIGHT 1977; WRIGHT et al. 1989). They concluded that "Physicians should be aware of the possibility that patients with ONSM may also harbor NF2." (BOSCH et al. 2006).

It is interesting that approximately 60% of sporadic meningiomas are caused by inactivation of NF2 suppressor gene on chromosome 2. There also appears to be a significant relationship between NF2 gene status, histologic subtype and anatomic tumor location (VAN TILBORG et al. 2005).

3.4.3
Bilateral Optic Nerve Sheath Meningioma

Dutton found 40 of 477 (8%) reported ONSM to be confined to the optic canal, with a high incidence of bilaterality (38%) compared to other locations. Some bilateral ONSM represent true, de-novo, multiple, independent tumors, but others are associated with neurofibromatosis type 2. The true incidence of bilateral isolated ONSM is difficult to estimate and most cases represent spread of tumor anteriorly into both optic canals from more posterior structures (TROBE et al. 1978). KENNERDELL and MAROON (1975) discuss a similar case defined at surgery with an intraorbital ONSM extending through the ipsilateral canal, across planum sphenoidale, and stopping just at the contralateral intracranial optic canal opening. Rootman describes half of the patients in his series with bilateral ONSM to have radiographic involvement of the planum sphenoidale in continuity with both optic canals (Saeed et al. 2003; Rootman 2003). The spread of an initially unilateral primary ONSM across to the contralateral optic nerve is rare.

3.4.4
Optic Nerve Sheath Meningioma in Pregnancy

Growth of ONSM may be initiated or accelerated in pregnancy. In some cases, a rapid growth phase is observed during pregnancy probably mediated by estrogen, progesterone, or androgen receptors. As in other forms of meningioma, stable, known, or occult ONSMs may exhibit accelerated growth and cause visual decline during pregnancy (Newell and Beamon 1958; Wan et al. 1990; Maxwell et al. 1993; Turbin et al. 2002; Wright 1977).

3.4.5
Optic Nerve Sheath Meningioma in Children

It has been reported that ONSM in children run a more aggressive clinical course, occasionally requiring complete surgical excision or exenteration (Alper 1981; Wright 1977; Wright et al. 1989; Ito et al. 1988; Jakobiec et al. 1984; Walsh 1970). Although possibly

more aggressive, Dutton concluded that there was little evidence to support that contralateral visual morbidity or patient mortality was at higher risk in these pediatric ONSM. Although five deaths were reported in cases of pediatric ONSM, all were related to operative complications or other causes (Alper 1981). In children it may be difficult to differentiate the more common optic nerve glioma from optic nerve sheath meningioma, and there are no completely valid clinical criteria (Karp et al. 1974). The entire clinical and radiographic picture must be considered, with occasional resort to incisional or excisional biopsy. Irregular nodular surface, calcification, and bone change (hyperostosis) are more common in ONSM, but imaging overlap occurs. Glioma may also be associated with arachnoid hyperplasia that may simulate ONSM (Fig. 3.14). Although the numbers are exceedingly small, the mean age of onset for five patients with bilateral ONSM was 12.8 years, suggesting a predominance in children (Dutton 1992).

3.4.6
Ectopic Intraorbital Meningioma

Dutton reviewed the concept of intraorbital meningioma arising from a site ectopic to the optic nerve sheath. He found an incidence of 4% primary ectopic orbital meningioma similar to Rootman's citation of 1 case in 23 (4%) (Table 3.1). Dutton concluded that the existence of true intraorbital ectopic meningioma is

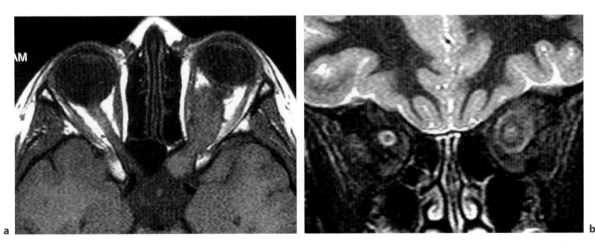

a   b

Fig. 3.14. a,b Fusiform enlargement and kinking of left optic nerve extending from left globe, up to and involving optic chiasm as shown on T1 axial image without fat suppression. Kinking, and intrinsic neural enlargement suggest glioma over meningioma. The T2 coronal image demonstrates fusiform enlargement of optic nerve glioma associated with concentric arachnoid hyperplasia, leading to an appearance that simulates ONSM in this case of biopsy proven (resection) glioma in a 12-year-old girl with neurofibromatosis 1. Similarly, some patients presumed to harbor optic nerve glioma are diagnosed with ONSM at time of surgery. **c** *see next page*

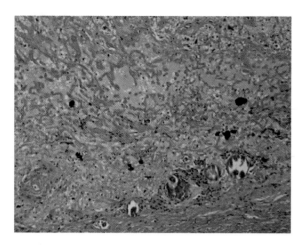

Fig. 3.14. (*continued*) **c** Hematoxylin and eosin preparation of meningothelial proliferation with microcystic spaces and calcification. Other sections of nerve showed true Rosenthal fibers c/w optic nerve glioma with reactive meningothelial hyperplasia in a 12-year-old girl with NF 1 (see **a,b**). *Courtesy of Paul Langer, MD and Neena Mirani, MD

open to debate, but probably represents a real but rare entity. We have not seen a true case at our institution. Authors have argued that these lesions might arise form orbital mesenchymal cells, represent extensions of arachnoid tufts from the optic nerve, or simply may represent misdiagnosis of other lesions (Karp et al. 1974; Spencer 1972; Shuanshoti 1973; Tan 1989). We have treated patients initially diagnosed with ectopic meningioma, whose lesions were reclassified as other entities by immunohistochemical analysis after recurrence.

3.5
Differential Diagnosis

Optic nerve glioma and meningioma are the commonest neoplasms affecting the optic nerve and may have overlapping features, although clinical differences separate the two lesions (Cooling and Wright 1979). For instance, some children thought to harbor optic nerve glioma may have ONSM, especially in patients with NF1 and concentric arachnoid hyperplasia (Fig. 3.14). The clinical presentation of ONSM may occasionally be difficult to distinguish from papillitis, perineuritis, sarcoid, unilateral papilledema, diabetic papillopathy, non arteritic ischemic optic neuropathy (NAION), leukemic

infiltrate, nonspecific orbital inflammation (NSOI) or other orbital tumors (Fig. 3.15). Orbital 2D B mode ultrasound may occasional be helpful to prove that a large orbital mass is distinct from the intraorbital optic nerve (Fig. 3.16). MRI and CT characteristics of ONSM are presented elsewhere in this text.

Continued visual loss despite the resolution of disc swelling in presumed NAION, progressive visual loss in "unobserved NAION" after disc edema resolution and cases mislabeled posterior ischemic optic neuropathy may harbor occult ONSM. However, in most of these cases chronic progressive visual loss is the rule and diagnosis is reached when visual loss progresses and patients are re-imaged with appropriate fat-suppressed gadolinium enhanced techniques. Sarcoid optic nerve involvement (neurosarcoid) is especially difficult to distinguish from some cases of ONSM (Figs. 3.17 and 3.18). The difficulty in distinguishing ONSM from sarcoid and other forms of inflammatory neuritis and perineuritis supports treatment with short empiric trials of high dose corticosteroids in patients with atypical radiographic findings or unexpected progressive visual loss and no other systemic or infectious contraindications. Indications and procedures for confirmatory biopsy will be discussed in a subsequent chapter.

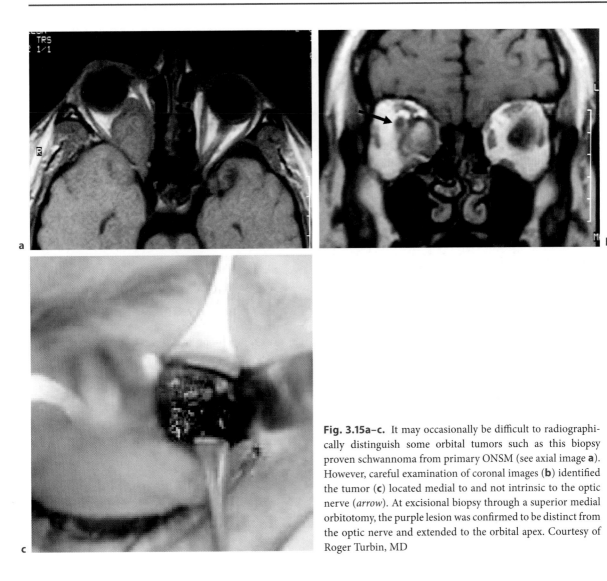

Fig. 3.15a–c. It may occasionally be difficult to radiographically distinguish some orbital tumors such as this biopsy proven schwannoma from primary ONSM (see axial image **a**). However, careful examination of coronal images (**b**) identified the tumor (**c**) located medial to and not intrinsic to the optic nerve (*arrow*). At excisional biopsy through a superior medial orbitotomy, the purple lesion was confirmed to be distinct from the optic nerve and extended to the orbital apex. Courtesy of Roger Turbin, MD

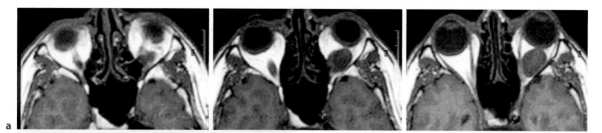

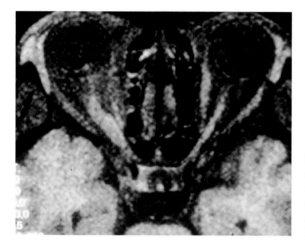

Fig. 3.16. Axial MRI images (**a**) without fat suppression fail to distinguish a large left orbital mass from the intraorbital optic nerve. However, 2D B scan ultrasound (**b**) delineates tumor (*white oval*) from optic nerve shadow (*white arrow*). Courtesy of Roger Turbin, MD

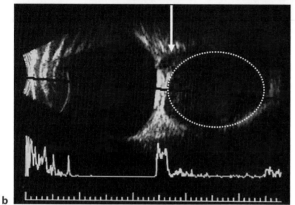

Fig. 3.17. T1 weighted fat suppressed axial image of right optic nerve lesion mimicking an apical and intraorbital tubular ONSM. Biopsy of this lesion ultimately revealed sarcoid. Sarcoid may be indistinguishable to even the most experienced clinicians and radiologists. Courtesy of Larry Frohman, MD

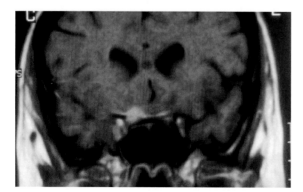

Fig. 3.18. Biopsy proven case of sarcoid simulating and orbital apex meningioma with intracranial extension, on T1 weighted coronal MRI. Courtesy of Larry Frohman, MD

A Suggested Approach to Clinical Evaluation

Unfortunately, there is no "magic" bullet to identify the subtle ONSM, although a high quality MRI with orbital fat suppression and gadolinium contrast nears the target. However, ONSM is a rare tumor and purchasing a neuroimaging study for all cases of optic neuropathy is neither cost efficient, safe, nor an effective practice of medicine. Few cases present with the classic triad, and other forms of optic atrophy may be indistinguishable on clinical grounds in more subtle cases. Yet the clinician is charged with appropriate identification and diagnosis of these lesions prior to the occurrence of irreversible visual loss. The physician, therefore, must develop a protocol to effectively sort out high risk presentations of optic neuropathy from more indolent forms. Again, because ONSM is a very uncommon entity, defining these strategies will serve the physician well and may even be more relevant to identification of many other progressive optic neuropathies. I strongly believe that the clinician is *not* always required to identify and diagnose ONSM at first clinical presentation given the similarity in presentation in most cases to other more "mundane" and more common forms of optic neuropathy. The clinician *is* charged with identifying and ultimately diagnosing these cases early as patients begin to manifest continued and progressive visual dysfunction. It is the follow-up, therefore, that is key to differentiating these clinical entities in cases that are not "obvious."

3.6.1
History

With few exceptions, most cases of sudden, severe, or painful visual loss that result in urgent patient visits are not related to primary ONSM. This generalization may not apply during pregnancy, in which more fulminant or even painful visual loss simulating optic neuritis occurs, although remains exceedingly uncommon. ONSM cases are typically identified after numerous clinical visits, previous non-diagnostic imaging studies, or failed surgical interventions. I have seen a number of patients who failed to improve after cataract extraction (with misidentification of underlying optic neuropathy), or who developed progressive visual loss after optic nerve pallor was incorrectly attributed to the assumption of past "unobserved" disc swelling. On the other hand, optic neuritis, non-arteritic ischemic optic neuropathy, arteritic ischemic optic neuropathy, inflammatory or autoimmune optic neuropathy are each very much

more common causes of an optic neuropathy, a pale, or a swollen optic nerve in appropriate age groups. Each of these potential mimics therefore requires appropriate historical support, demonstration of typical clinical course, or confirmation of absence of compressive intracranial lesion on clinical or radiographic grounds. Appropriate history, review of symptoms, and identification of systemic disease known to be risk factors to these more common entities is therefore time consuming but imperative. The pale or chronically swollen optic nerve associated with worsening visual function or subacute progressive visual loss must be identified, and requires further evaluation as it may harbor the unexpected compressive, inflammatory, or infiltrative lesion.

3.6.2
Physical Examination

The physical examination in patients identified to manifest an optic neuropathy should be painstakingly empiric, quantifying current level of function to provide benchmarks for future identification of potential visual loss. A careful, complete ophthalmologic examination is in order, as in all cases of optic neuropathy, and should quantify best potential corrected visual acuity, kinetic or static visual field testing, color vision testing, pupil testing, tonometry, as well as all components of a slit lamp biomicroscopic and fundoscopic examination, including optic nerve head appearance and presence or absence of nerve fiber layer loss. Ocular motility testing, prism measurement of ocular misalignment, exophthalmometry, detection of resistance to ocular retropulsion and assessment of cranial nerve testing are all germane. There is simply no substitute for an accurate, quantitative, complete examination. Precise assessment of visual acuity is especially important. The notation "finger counting" is imprecise, and a more quantitative angular assessment such as 20/800, 20/1000, etc. provides more information for future evaluation. Similarly, the measure of the depth of relative afferent pupil with neutral density filters may provide a baseline for future comparison, and is a cost effective, rapid, and efficient alternative to pupillography which is currently primarily available only as a research technique.

3.6.3
Ancillary Testing

Ophthalmology and radiology are technologically driven fields, and continuous advancements in imaging capability and resolution lend difficulty to review adequately all available testing and the application to ONSM. Similarly, the low incidence of ONSM make it unlikely that future studies will be performed that directly assess utility of myriads of new clinical techniques. Yet, advances in medicine as a field have paralleled advances in imaging and we continue to learn as we delve into deeper levels of structural-functional correlation. I have made it my practice to apply Jack Kennerdell's wisdom in reassessing and applying developing technologies that increasingly define structural and functional detail.

As such, advances in ophthalmic imaging of nerve fiber layer (retinal photography, optical coherence tomography scanning laser polarimetry, and confocal laser scanning) may help identify progressive structural loss of nerve fiber layer and contribute to medical decision making as well as the decision to institute treatment of ONSM. Fluroscein angiography has a role in selected cases and may help differentiate the etiology of choroidal–retinal shunt vessels in compressive cases from vascular causes. Optic nerve ultrasonograpy is portable, readily available, and may identify an optic nerve lesion that signals the need for more advanced neuroimaging.

In appropriate clinical scenarios, additional ancillary testing is directed toward the identification of concurrent disease that may produce a lesion that radiographically mimics ONSM. Sarcoid optic neuropathy and syphilitic perineuritis, among a number of other uncommon inflammatory, infectious, infiltrative, autoimmune, or neoplastic lesions are probably the most common mimics in adults in our clinics. We have outlined our clinical approach to the diagnosis of sarcoid disease elsewhere, but frequently employ gallium citrate full body and positron emission tomography (PET) full body imaging to identify areas of radiographic abnormality outside of the orbit that may be more amenable to safe biopsy and confirm nocaseating granulomatous disease (FROHMAN et al. 2003). Similarly, we frequently assess CSF pressure, chemistry and cellular makeup, as well as syphilitic serology.

3.6.4
Ordering Radiographic Images

High quality, high resolution gadolinium contrast enhanced, fat suppressed MRI imaging of the orbit (which typically overlaps appropriate intracranial structures and may alleviate the need for a separate brain study) is a mainstay in diagnosis and subsequent follow-up of ONSM in our clinics. It is important that the clinician be familiar with the limitations and quality of a given scan and the scanner from which it is derived, and must review studies in radiographic consultation to ensure that appropriate high field techniques (1.5 tesla and above) without confounding artifact (especially failure of fat suppression or movement artifact) are available. Although prior studies may truly be negative in patients harboring an occult ONSM, it is our experience that initial studies were more frequently misread, or of inadequate quality.

High quality, thin cut (1.0–1.5 mm) computed tomography of the orbit evaluated in axial and coronal views before and after contrast injection may also be useful in selected cases. CT in some centers may be more available, rapidly performed (therefore less susceptible to movement artifact), less expensive, and more sensitive to the calcium in some lesions. In addition, size, weight, claustrophobic tendencies, and presence of paramagnetic foreign bodies may preclude some patients from having MRI. Authors have recently described the utility of functional 111 In-octreotide single-photon emission computed tomography as an adjunct to MRI in assessing ONSM clinical disease activity, but we have limited experience with this clinical application (ANDREWS et al. 2002). The specific imaging criteria for diagnosis of ONSM are detailed elsewhere in this text.

3.6.5
Medical Decision Making

A key to diagnosis is the transition in thought process as to when a particular optic neuropathy becomes "atypical" or progressive. The majority of patients with optic neuropathy in our clinic represent "run of the mill" demyelinating or post-infectious optic neuritis in children or younger and middle-aged adults, and ischemic non-arteritic or arteritic optic neuropathy in the more mature population. The former patients typically undergo MRI imaging at baseline and the latter do not. Patients who fail to respond to corticosteroid therapy or recur after corticosteroid taper and patients who progress in the subacute period (months to years after an event) are atypical and demand additional thoughtful evaluation. Some patients previously diagnosed with an enhancing optic nerve-sheath complex identified to be consistent with optic neuritis will later be recognized to harbor ONSM or other inflammatory or infiltrative causes of a perineuritis. Similarly, patients who manifest persistent or progressive unilateral optic nerve head edema not attributed to other causes after months of observation are suspect. On the other hand, patients who have not undergone biopsy and have lesions presumed to be ONSM based on clinical course and radiographic appearance may harbor other lesions (see Sect. 3.2.2).

Occasionally, the physician is faced with significant clinical uncertainty based on atypical appearance, clinical or radiographic progression. If additional testing fails to identify concurrent telltale disease the clinician may be forced by clinical uncertainty to utilize a brief corticosteroid trial or resort to a conservative, limited biopsy. Indications for surgery are addressed in a subsequent chapter.

References

Alper MG (1981) Management of primary optic nerve meningiomas. J Clin Neuro-ophthalmol 1:101–117

Alper MG, Sherman JL (1989) Gadolinium enhanced magnetic resonance imaging in the diagnosis of anterior visual pathway meningiomas. Trans Am Ophthalmol Soc 87:384–419

Als E (1969) Intraorbital meningiomas encasing the optic nerve. Acta Ophthalmol 47:900–903

Amoli FA, Mehrabani PM, Tari AS (2007) Aggressive orbital optic nerve meningioma with benign microscopic features: a case report. Orbit 26(4):271–274

Andrews DW, Faroozan R, Yang BP (2002) Fractionated stereotactic radiotherapy for the treatment of optic nerve sheath meningiomas: preliminary observations of 33 optic nerves in 30 patients with historical comparison to observation with or without prior surgery. Neurosurgery 51(4):890–902

Becker G, Jeremic B, Pitz S et al. (2002) Stereotactic fractionated radiotherapy in patients with optic nerve sheath meningioma. Int J Radiat Oncol Biol Phys 54(5):1422–1429

Bosch MM, Wichmann WW, Boltshauser E, Landau K (2006) Optic nerve sheath meningiomas in patients with neurofibromatosis type 2. Arch Ophthalmol 124(3):379–385

Castel A, Boschi A, Renard L et al. (2000) Optic nerve sheath meningiomas: clinical features, functional prognosis and controversial treatment. Bull Soc Belge Ophtalmol 275:73–78

Cibis GW, Whittaker CK, Wood WE (1985) Intraocular extension of optic nerve meningioma in a case of neurofibromatosis. Arch Ophthalmol 103:404–406

Clark WC, Theofilos CS, Fleming JC (1989) Primary optic nerve sheath meningiomas. Report of nine cases. J Neurosurg 70:37–40

Cooling RJ, Wright JE (1979) Arachnoid hyperplasia in optic nerve glioma: confusion with orbital meningioma. Br J Ophthalmol 63(9):596–599

Coston T (1936) Primary tumor of the optic nerve. With a report of a case. Arch Ophthalmol 15:696–702

Créange A, Zeller J, Rostaing-Rigattieri S et al. (1999) Neurological complications of neurofibromatosis type 1 in adulthood. Brain 122:473–481

Cristante L (1994) Surgical treatment of meningiomas of the orbit and optic canal: a retrospective study with particular attention to the visual outcome. Acta Neurochir (Wien) 126(1):27–32

Cunliffe IA, Moffat DA, Hardy DG, Moore AT (1992) Bilateral optic nerve sheath meningiomas in a patient with neurofibromatosis type 2. Br J Ophthalmol 76:310–312

Cushing H, Eisenhardt L (1938) Meningiomas: their classification, regional behavior, life history and surgical end results. Charles C. Thomas, Springfield, Ill, pp 250–282

Dutton JJ (1992) Optic nerve sheath meningiomas. Surv Ophthalmol 37(3):167–183

Egan RA, Lessell S (2002) A contribution to the natural history of optic nerve sheath meningiomas. Arch Ophthalmol 120(11):1505–1508

Elschnig A (1898) Ueber opticociliare Gefasse. Klin Mbl Augenheilk 36:93–96

Evans DG, Moran A, King A et al. (2005) Incidence of vestibular schwannoma and neurofibromatosis 2 in the North West of England over a 10-year period: higher incidence than previously thought. Otolol Neurotol 26(1):93–97

Frasier BS, Green RL (2002) Ultrasound of the eye and orbit, 2nd edn. Mosby, St. Louis, p 424

Frisen L, Hoyt WF, Tengroth BM (1973) Optociliary veins, disc pallor and visual loss: a triad of signs indicating sphenoorbital meningioma. Acta Ophthalmol 51:241–249

Frohman LP, Guirgis M, Turbin RE, Bielory L (2003) Sarcoidosis of the anterior visual pathway: 24 new cases. J Neuro-Ophthalmol 23(3):190–197

Hartmann E (1933) Enlargissement du canal optique visible à la radiographie chez les malades atteints de neurofibromatose avec tumeur du nerf optique. J Belge Neurol Psychiatr 33:763–772

Hirst LW, Miller NR, Allen GS (1979) Sphenoidal pneumosinus dilatans with bilateral optic nerve meningiomas. Case report. J Neurosurg 51(3):402–407

Imes RK, Schatz H, Hoyt WF et al. (1985) Evolution of optociliary veins in optic nerve sheath meningioma. Arch Ophthalmol 103(1):59–60

Ito M, Ishizawa A, Miyaoka M et al. (1988) Intraorbital meningiomas: surgical management and role of radiation therapy. Surg Neurol 29:448–453

Jackson A, Patankara T, Laitt L (2003) Intracanalicular optic nerve meningioma: a serious diagnostic pitfall. Am J Neuroradiol 24:1167–1170

Jakobiec FA, Depot MJ, Kennerdell JS et al. (1984) Combined clinical and computed tomographic diagnosis of orbital glioma and meningioma. Ophthalmology 1:137–155

Karp LA, Zimmerman LE, Borit A et al. (1974) Primary intraorbital meningioma. Arch Ophthalmol 91:24–28

Kennerdell JS, Maroon JC (1975) Intracanalicular meningioma with chronic optic disc edema. Ann Ophthalmol 7(4):507–512

Kondziolka D, Mathieu D, Lunsford LD et al. (2008) Radiosurgery as definitive management of intracranial meningiomas. Neurosurgery 62(1):53–58

Laitt RD, Kumar B, Leatherbarrow B et al. (1996) Cystic optic nerve meningioma presenting with acute proptosis. Eye 10:744–746

Larson JJ, van Loveren HR, Balko MG, Tew JM Jr (1995) Evidence of meningioma infiltration into cranial nerves: clinical implications for cavernous sinus meningiomas. J Neurosurg 83(4):596–599

Lindblom B, Norman D, Hoyt WF (1992a) Perioptic cyst distal to optic nerve meningioma: MR demonstration. Am J Neuroradiol 13(6):1622–1624

Lindblom B, Truwit CL, Hoyt WF (1992b) Optic nerve sheath meningioma. Definition of intraorbital, intracanalicular, and intracranial components with magnetic resonance imaging. Ophthalmology 99(4):560–566

Mathiesen T, Kihlström L (2006) Visual outcome of tuberculum sellae meningiomas after extradural optic nerve decompression. Neurosurgery 59(3):570–576

Maxwell M, Galanopoulos T, Neville-Golden J et al. (1993) Expression of androgen and progesterone receptors in primary human meningiomas. J Neurosurg 78:456–462

McNab AA, Wright JE (1989) Cysts of the optic nerve. Three cases associated with meningioma. Eye 3:355–359

Mehra KS, Khanna SS, Dube B (1979) Primary meningioma of the intraorbital optic nerve. Ann Ophthalmol 11(5):758–760

Miller NR (2006) New concepts in the diagnosis and management of optic nerve sheath meningioma. J Neuroophthalmol 26(3):200–208

Miller NR, Golnik KC, Zeidman SM et al. (1996) Pneumosinus dilatans: a sign of intracranial meningioma. Surg Neurol 46(5):471–474

Newell FW, Beamon TC (1958) Ocular signs of meningiomas. Am J Ophthalmol 45:30–40

Ortiz O, Schochet SS, Kotzan JM et al. (1996) Radiologic-pathologic correlation: meningioma of the optic nerve sheath. Am J Neuroradiol 17(5):901–906

Parker H (1922) A case of von Recklinghausen's disease with involvement of the peripheral nerves, optic nerve and spinal cord. J Nerv Ment Dis 56:441–452

Peele KA, Kennerdell JS, Maroon JC et al. (1996) The role of postoperative irradiation in the management of sphenoid wing meningiomas. A preliminary report. Ophthalmology 103(11):1761–1766

Probst C, Gessaga E, Leuenberger AE (1985) Primary meningioma of the optic nerve sheaths: case report. Ophthalmologica 190(2):83–90

Ringel F, Cedzich C, Schramm J (2007) Microsurgical technique and results of a series of 63 spheno-orbital meningiomas. Neurosurgery 60(4 Suppl 2):214–221

Rootman J (2003) Diseases of the orbit. A multidisciplinary approach, 2nd edn. Lipincott Williams & Wilkins, Philadelphia, pp 232–240

Rosca TI, Carstocea BD, Vlădescu TG et al. (2006) Cystic optic nerve sheath meningioma. J Neuroophthalmol 26(2):121–122

Saeed P, Rootman J, Nugent RA et al. (2003) Optic nerve sheath meningiomas. Ophthalmology 110(10):2019–2030

Salzmann M (1893) Zur Anatomie der angeborenen Sichel nach innen-unten. Albrecht von Grefes Arch Ophtal 39:131–150

Schick U, Hassler W (2005) Surgical management of tuberculum sellae meningiomas: involvement of the optic canal and visual outcome. J Neurol Neurosurg Psychiatry 76(7):977–983

Schittkowski M, Hingst V, Stropahl G et al. (1999) Optic nerve sheath meningioma with intraocular invasion–a case report. Klin Monatsbl Augenheilkd 214(4):251–254

Sen C, Hague K (1997) Meningiomas involving the cavernous sinus: histological factors affecting the degree of resection. J Neurosurg 87(4):535–543

Shapland CD, Greenfield JG (1935) Case of neurofibromatosis with meningeal tumor involving left optic nerve. Trans Ophthalmol Soc U K 55:257–279

Shuanshoti S (1973) Meningioma of the optic nerve. Br J Ophthalmol 57(4):265–269

Spencer W (1972) Primary neoplasms of the optic nerve and its sheaths: clinical features and current concepts of the pathogenetic mechanisms. Trans AM Ophthalmol Soc 70:490–528

Susac JO, Smith JL, Walsh FB (1977) The impossible meningioma. Arch Neurol 34:36–38

Swenson SA, Forbes GS, Younge BR, Campbell RJ (1982) Radiologic evaluation of tumors of the optic nerve. Am J Neuroradiol 3:319–326

Tan FL (1989) CT scan and clinical diagnosis of parasellar lesions – analysis of 91 cases. Zhonghua Zhong Liu Za Zhi 11(4):291–293

Trobe JD, Glaser JS, Post JD, Page LK (1978) Bilateral optic canal meningiomas: a case report. Neurosurgery 3(1):68–74

Trobe JD, Glaser JS, Cassady JC (1980) Optic atrophy. Differential diagnosis by fundus observation alone. Arch Ophthalmol 98(6):1040–1045

Turbin RE, Pokorny K (2004) Diagnosis and treatment of orbital optic nerve sheath meningioma. Cancer Control 11(5):334–341

Turbin RE, Thompson CR, Kennerdell JS, Cockerham KP, Kupersmith MJ (2002) A long-term visual outcome comparison in patients with optic nerve sheath meningioma managed with observation, surgery, radiotherapy, or surgery and radiotherapy. Ophthalmology 109(5):890–899

Turbin RE, Wladis EJ, Frohman LP et al. (2006) Role for surgery as adjuvant therapy in optic nerve sheath meningioma. Ophthal Plast Reconstr Surg 22(4):278–282

van Tilborg AA, Al Allak B, Velthuize SC et al. (2005) Chromosomal instability in meningiomas. J Neuropathol Exp Neurol 64(4):312–322

Walsh F (1970) Meningiomas primary within the orbit and optic canal. In: Smith JL (ed) Neuro-ophthalmology Symposium of the University of Miami and the Bascom Palmer Eye Institute. Mosby, St Louis, Mo, pp 240–266

Wan WL, Geller JL, Feldon SE et al. (1990) Visual loss caused by rapidly progressive intracranial meningiomas during pregnancy. Ophthalmology 97:18–21

Worster-Drought C, Dickson WEC, McMenemey WH (1937) Multiple meningeal and perineural tumors with analogous changes in the glia and ependyma (neurofibroblastomatosis), with report of two cases. Brain 60:85–117

Wright JE (1977) Primary optic nerve meningiomas: clinical presentation and management. Trans Am Acad Opthalmol Otolaryngol 83:617–625

Wright JE, McNab AA, McDonald WI (1989) Primary optic nerve sheath meningioma. Br J Ophthalmol 73:960–966

Imaging Diagnosis of the Optic Nerve Sheath Meningioma

Mahmood F. Mafee and John H. Naheedy

CONTENTS

KEY POINTS

Optic nerve sheath meningiomas classically are seen in middle-aged or elderly females and present as slowly progressing axial proptosis and gradual loss of vision. In addition to the appropriate clinical presentation, the diagnosis of optic nerve sheath tumors falls heavily on the imaging findings, especially given the complexity of their location and the considerable morbidities that may be associated with biopsy. Cross-sectional imaging is an essential diagnostic tool and magnetic resonance (MR) imaging in particular, with the increasing clinical availability of 3-Tesla magnets, remains the modality of choice for the imaging diagnosis of optic nerve pathology. Computed tomography (CT), however, is not without its advantages and can often reveal characteristic findings to help make the diagnosis. Thus, knowledge of the MR and CT imaging characteristics of optic nerve sheath meningiomas, in conjunction with a suitable clinical context, is essential to accurate diagnosis and differentiation from other similar appearing lesions.

M. F. Mafee, MD, FACR
Professor of Clinical Radiology, Vice Chair for Education, Residency Program Director, UCSD Medical Center, 200 West Arbor Drive, San Diego, CA 92103, USA

J. H. Naheedy, MD
Chief Resident, Department of Radiology, University of California, San Diego, 200 West Arbor Drive, San Diego, CA 92103-8756, USA

4.1
Introduction

Optic nerve meningiomas arise from the meningothelial cells of the arachnoid membrane that are situated along the optic nerve sheath. Thus, in order to study this lesion best, one requires a full understanding of the meninges themselves. The dura mater (from the Latin "hard mother"), is described as having two layers, the outer (endosteal) layer and the inner meningeal layer (dura mater proper).

The outer *endosteal layer* is the functional periosteum, covering the inner surface of the skull bones. It is tightly adherent to the skull bone and becomes continuous with the periosteum on the outside of the skull bones (MAFEE 2005a; MAFEE et al. 2005) around the margins of the skull base foramina/fissures as well as the optic canal where it is most strongly adherent to the osseous structures (SNELL and LAMP 1989).

The inner meningeal layer is a dense fibrous membrane covering the brain and is continuous through the foramen magnum with the dura mater of the spinal cord (unlike the endosteal layer that fuses at the foramen magnum). Inside the skull the meningeal layer provides tubular sheaths for the cranial nerves as it passes through the foramina in the skull. Outside of the skull the meningeal layer fuses with the perineurium of the cranial nerves. The meningeal layer of the dura is firmly attached to the outer (periosteal) layer; however, at the optic canal, it becomes separated from the outer layer and forms a dural sleeve for the optic nerve. This dural sleeve extends along the optic nerve and forms the outer wall of the subarachnoid space surrounding the optic nerve, later fusing at the globe (tenon capsule).

Understanding the anatomy of the meninges and ophthalmic artery as it relates to the orbit is also essential to the analysis of imaging findings and particularly to the surgical approach. The ophthalmic artery is intradural in the optic canal and then its branches cross the subarachnoid space to surround the optic nerve, carrying with them dura-derived fibrous tissue. This intimate relationship of the blood supply to the optic nerve and the meninges is probably the reason why surgical intervention in which the dura is manipulated and incised so often deprives optic nerve of blood supply and blinds the involved eye (MAFEE et al. 1999b; WALSH 1975).

Similarly, knowledge of the histology of the arachnoid membrane outer layer and inner layer is important in understanding the histologic classification of varied histopathological meningioma subtypes: meningothelial, fibroblastic, and transitional. The outer layer of the arachnoid membrane, composed of epithelial – type cells, consists of numerous tightly packed cells and is thought to give rise to cellular types of meningiomas. The subarachnoid space contains cerebrospinal fluid (CSF), blood vessels and arachnoid trabeculae, which are cores of fibrous tissue surrounded by mesothelium. The arachnoid trabeculae are thought to give rise to angioblastic or lipoblastic meningiomas. The inner layer of the arachnoid membrane consists of stratified fibrous tissue, giving rise to mixed or fibromatous meningiomas (MAFEE et al. 1999b; WALSH 1975).

4.2
Clinical Presentation

Optic nerve sheath meningiomas are rare tumors and comprise approximately 2% of all orbital tumors and 1%–2% of all meningiomas (EDDLEMAN and LIU 2007). The classic clinical presentation consists of slowly progressive, painless visual loss. On clinical examination, axial proptosis (GREENBERG 1998; JACOBIEC et al. 1984; MILLER 2006) and the presence of optocilliary venous shunts on the disk (when accompanied by disk pallor and visual loss) is highly suggestive of an indolent nerve sheath meningioma (MAFEE et al. 1992; LLOYD 1982). The demographic distribution of 2:1 women to men is attributable to the presence of progesterone receptor mRNA expression on most meningiomas (MAFEE et al. 1999b).

The majority of optic nerve sheath meningioma arises either from the meningothelial cells of the arachnoid that are situated along the optic nerve sheath. However, a subset of optic nerve sheath meningiomas arise from extension of an intracranial meningioma (spheno-orbital meningiomas) into the orbit. Another rare group (extradural meningioma) consists of tumors arising from ectopic arachnoid cells within the orbit.

4.3
Imaging Features

Given the complexity of their location and the considerable morbidities that may be associated with biopsy, diagnosis of optic nerve sheath tumors falls heavily on imaging findings, in addition to the clinical presentation (TURBIN and POKORNY 2004; MILLER 2006). On plain film radiography, optic nerve sheath meningiomas characteristically give little sign of their presence; although, in later stages of disease enlargement or hyperostosis of the optic canal can sometime be appreciated. Rather, it is computed tomography (CT) and magnetic resonance (MR) which are the foundation for imaging diagnosis (MAFEE 1992, 1996a, b; LLOYD 1982; LEE et al. 1997; WEBER et al. 1996; MOUTON et al. 2007).

4.3.1
Computed Tomography Imaging

CT is an excellent imaging study for evaluating optic nerve sheath meningioma, particularly when performed

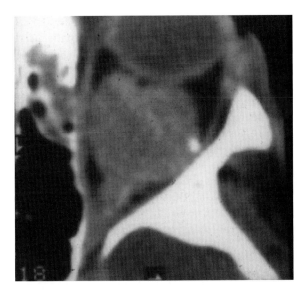

Fig. 4.1. Optic nerve sheath meningioma. Enhanced axial CT image, shows moderately enhancing mass with calcification around the optic nerve

both before and after intravenous infusion of iodinated-based contrast medium. Thin sections (1.5–3 mm) are essential to visualize the tumor, its actual extent and the presence of micro/macro calcifications. As previously discussed, given its intimate association with the dura mater, optic nerve sheath meningiomas often appear as a well defined, tubular or fusiform thickening of the optic nerve (Fig. 4.1). Characteristic findings may include diffuse, tubular enlargement or localized, eccentric expansion of the optic nerve, and not uncommonly at the orbital apex. At times, small en plaque optic nerve sheath meningiomas may be best visualized by CT due to calcifications (Fig. 4.2).

Unenhanced CT scans, may demonstrate diffuse calcifications within or along an optic nerve sheath complex mass, either linear and plaquelike (placoid) or focal granular, which are highly suggestive of an optic nerve sheath meningioma (Fig. 4.3). At times a dense diffuse calcified optic nerve-sheath complex (with or

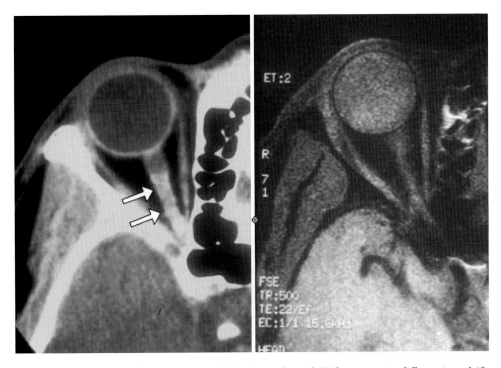

Fig. 4.2. Optic nerve sheath meningioma. *Left*: Axial unenhanced CT demonstrating diffuse microcalcifications around the optic nerve. *Right*: Axial enhanced fat saturation (FS) T1 weighted MR fails to demonstrate the lesion seen on CT

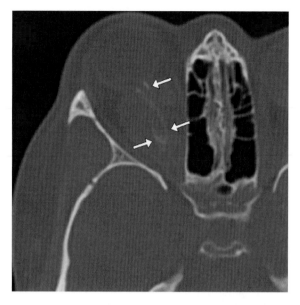

Fig. 4.3. Optic nerve sheath meningioma. Axial CT shows diffuse calcifications along the optic nerve sheath (*arrows*). The meningioma itself is seen as a fusiform mass surrounding the optic nerve

without focal or diffuse enlargement of the optic nerve) may be present. While calcification in meningiomas is not uncommon, in very rare instances, optic nerve gliomas may also demonstrate calcification. However, GREENBERG (1998) reported that idiopathic optic nerve sheath calcifications can indeed occur.

Post-contrast images typically show homogenous and well-defined contrast enhancement. The classic CT finding of a "Tram-Track" sign refers to the central lucency of the optic nerve pancaked between an enlarged and enhanced optic nerve-sheath complex. However, while this was originally described in optic nerve sheath meningiomas, it is not specific for this entity as it may also be seen in CT scans of pseudotumors, lymphoma, sarcoidosis, and leptomeningeal carcinomatosis. Meningiomas surround the optic nerve, and thus the caliber of the nerve itself is attenuated within the surrounding tumor. This is in contrast to the optic nerve gliomas, where the nerve itself appears expanded. This feature is best appreciated in coronal sections, particularly on MR images (Fig. 4.4).

Sphenoid pneumosinus dilatans is an additional CT sign that may be associated with intracanalicular optic nerve sheath meningiomas as well as spheno-orbital meningiomas (HIRST et al. 1982). The involved expanded sinus may be the ethmoid, sphenoid, or frontal-sinuses. However, this is relatively nonspecific

and at times may be seen in normal subjects. The CT appearance of pneumosinus dilatans in optic nerve sheath meningioma or periforaminal meningioma may be seen as an expanded ("blistering") posterior ethmoid air cell or a pneumatized anterior clinoid.

Less conventional imaging methods, such as CT cisternography, may also lead to diagnosis. Fox et al. (1979) reported a very unusual case of tiny meningioma, detected by intrathecal metrizamide cisternography. The tumor was subsequently removed with a return to normal vision of the previously blind eye. However, with the advent of MRI, even small optic nerve sheath meningiomas can be readily visualized without need for intrathecal contrast injection to perform CT cisternography.

4.3.2
Magnetic Resonance Imaging

Despite its decreased sensitivity for detecting calcification (relative to CT), magnetic resonance (MR) imaging remains the modality of choice for the imaging diagnosis of optic nerve sheath meningioma, spheno-orbital meningioma and other optic nerve pathologic conditions. On MR imaging, meningiomas can be seen as a localized (Fig. 4.5), diffuse or fusiform enlargement of the optic nerve sheath complex (Fig. 4.6) and may be eccentric (Fig. 4.7). The tumor retains an isointense appearance to the optic nerve and brain tissue on most MRI imaging pulse sequences (Fig. 4.4). The T1-weighted (T1W) and T2-weighted (T2W) MR images usually show no significant differences in signal intensity of meningiomas compared with that of the normal optic nerve or brain tissue. Compared with the brain, however, meningiomas may also be hypointense on T1W and proton-weighted (PW) MR images and hyperintense or even hypointense (depending on calcification or pact fibroblastic histologic feature) on T2W MR images.

Gadolinium-based contrast enhanced fat-suppression T1W pulse sequences have made a significant contribution to the orbital imaging and are widely considered the gold-standard examination for evaluation of disorders of the optic nerve (MOUTON et al. 2007). T1W MR images obtained following IV injection of the gadolinium-based contrast material demonstrate moderate to marked contrast enhancement of meningiomas (Figs. 4.4–4.7). Post contrast enhanced fat suppression T1W MR images are most valuable for defining and enhancing optic nerve pathology (Fig. 4.8).

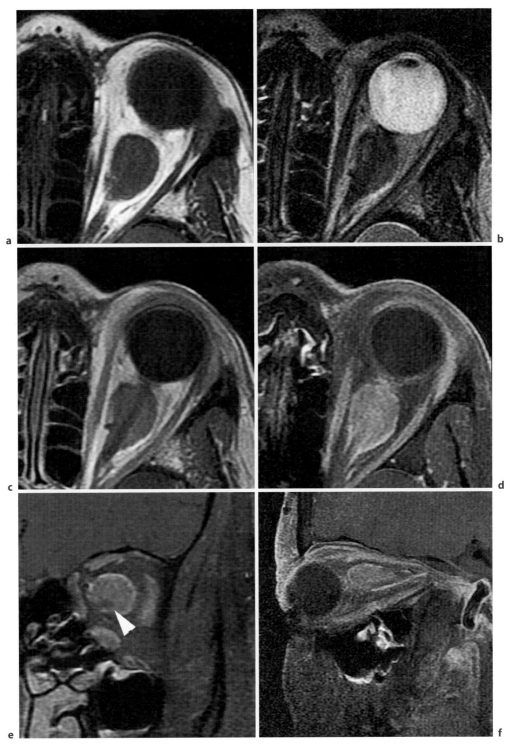

Fig. 4.4a–f. Optic nerve sheath menigioma on 3T magnet. **a** Unenhanced T1W. **b** Fast Spin Echo (FSE) T2W. **c** Enhanced T1W. **d** Enhanced fat suppression T1W. **e** Enhanced coronal fat suppression T1W. **f** Sagittal enhanced fat suppresion T1W. *Arrowhead* in **e** points out the optic nerve surrounded by the optic nerve sheath meningioma. Note in this case that the meningtioma is isointense to orbital muscles on the T1W and T2W images. (From: Mafee MF, Rapoport M, Karimi A, Ansari S, Shah J (2005) Orbital and ocular imaging using 3- and 1.5-T MR imaging systems. Neuroimag Clin N Am 15:4; with permission)

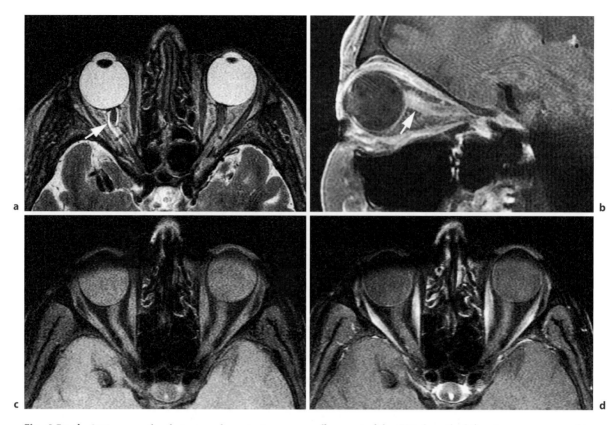

Fig. 4.5a–d. Optic nerve sheath presumed meningioma on 3T magnet. **a** Axial T2W. **b** Enhanced fat suppressed sagittal T1W. **c** Unenhanced fat suppressed axial T1W. **d** Enhanced fat suppressed axial T1W showing a left optic nerve sheath meningioma which is less well depicted on axial MR imaging and best demonstrated (*arrow* in **b**) on enhanced MR imaging. Note the effacement of the CSF along the left optic nerve compared to the contralateral normal. (From: Mafee MF, Rapoport M, Karimi A, Ansari S, Shah J (2005) Orbital and ocular imaging using 3- and 1.5-T MR imaging systems. Neuroimag Clin N Am 15:6; with permission)

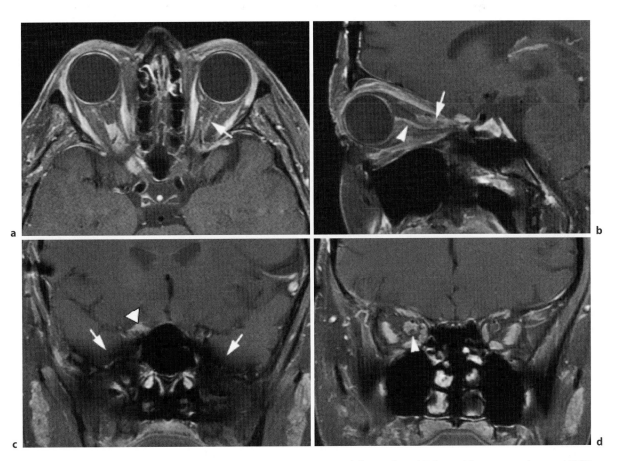

Fig. 4.6a–d. Optic nerve sheath meningioma on 3T magnet. **a** Enhanced fat suppressed axial T1W with diffuse enhancement of the right optic nerve sheath meningioma. Note the normal left optic nerve (*arrow*). **b** Enhanced fat suppressed sagittal T1W. **c** Enhanced fat suppressed coronal T1W showing the meningioma involving the intracranial segment of the right optic nerve (*wide arrowhead*). *Arrows* point out the magnetic susceptibility artifact. **d** Enhanced fat suppressed coronal T1W with the *arrowhead* depicting the constricted optic nerve surrounded by a optic nerve sheath meningioma. (From: Mafee MF, Rapoport M, Karimi A, Ansari S, Shah J (2005) Orbital and ocular imaging using 3- and 1.5-T MR imaging systems. Neuroimag Clin N Am 15:6; with permission)

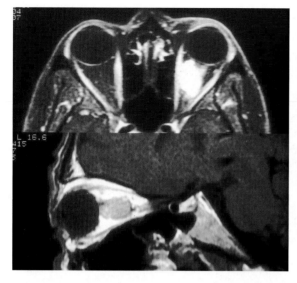

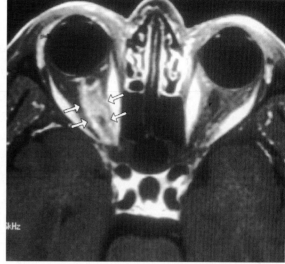

Fig. 4.7. Optic nerve sheath meningioma. Enhanced axial FS T1W (*top*) and enhanced sagittal non-fat saturation T1W (*bottom*) MR images demonstrate left optic nerve sheath meningioma with an exophytic pattern of growth

Fig. 4.8. *En plaque* meningioma. Enhanced fat suppressed axial T1W MR image shows *en plaque* meningioma along the right optic nerve (*arrows*)

4.4
Special Situations

Intracranial extension of optic nerve sheath meningiomas or intraorbital extension of an intracranial meningioma may easily be demonstrated on either post-contrast CT scans or enhanced T1W MR images. *En plaque* meningiomas of the optic nerve sheath, where the tumor spreads out along the optic nerve sheath as a thin or slightly thick tumor, can often only be diagnosed as abnormal enhancement of the optic nerve on enhanced fat suppression T1W MR images (Figs. 4.6 and 4.8). Intracanalicular optic meningiomas usually represent either extensions of posterior orbital tumors or invasion into the optic canal by periforaminal meningiomas arising in the vicinity of the anterior clinoid.

Childhood optic nerve sheath meningiomas are often associated with neurofibromatosis Type 2 (NF2) and are usually more aggressive than the adult form (Fig. 4.9) (BOSCH et al. 2006). Children have a higher recurrence rate and a poorer survival rate than adults (TURBIN and POKORNY 2004). Bilateral optic nerve sheath meningiomas may occur in patients with or without NF (Fig. 4.10) (JACOBIEC et al. 1984). Even neurofibromas, at times, may be mistaken on imaging

and histologic evaluation for optic nerve sheath meningiomas (Fig. 4.11).

Another rare group of meningiomas includes the ectopic, intraorbital, extradural meningiomas. These tumors do not appear to have any connection to the optic nerve sheath or the optic canal and do not appear to originate intracranially (MAFEE 1992). They arise from congenitally misplaced nests of ectopic meningothelial cells within the orbital cavity, either in the muscle cone or in the walls of the orbit. They are frequently associated with characteristic, localized expansion of adjacent ethmoid air cells, or so-called "blistering."

4.5
Differential Diagnosis
of Optic Nerve Enlargement

The finding of optic nerve enlargement may result from several different pathologic entities, including sarcoidosis (MAFEE et al. 1999a), lymphoma (MAFEE et al. 2005), optic glioma (HOLLANDER et al. 1999), pseudo-tumor and optic neuritis (MAFEE 2005a), which must be distinguished from optic nerve meningiomas to ensure optimal management. Sarcoidosis has a strong

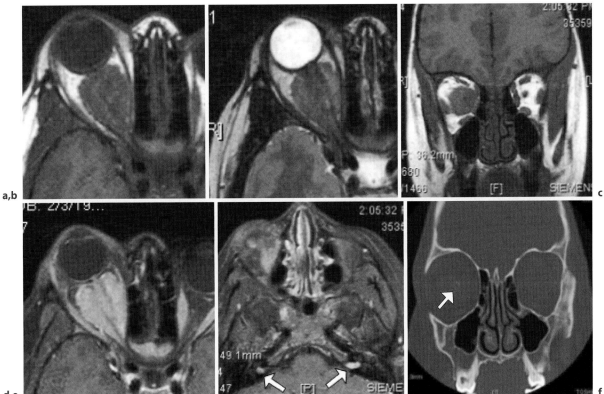

Fig. 4.9a–f. Optic nerve sheath meningioma. A 12-year-old male with neurofibromatosis type 2 and a large right optic nerve sheath meningioma. **a** Axial unenhanced T1W. **b** Axial T2W. **c** Coronal unenhanced T1W. **d** Axial enhanced FS T1W.

e Axial enhanced FS T1W MR images showing bilateral vestibular schwannomas (*arrows*). **f** Coronal CT with *arrow* pointing to right optic nerve sheath calcification.

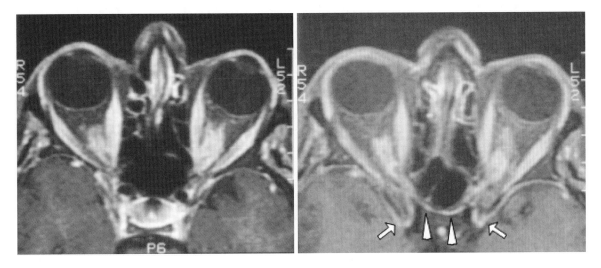

Fig. 4.10. Bilateral *en plaque* optic nerve sheath meningiomas. *Left*: Axial enhanced T1W fat suppressed MR showing abnormal enhancement of both optic nerves. *Right*: Note the abnormal dural enhancement along the chiasmatic sulcus (*arrows*) and along the anterior clinoids bilaterally (*arrowheads*)

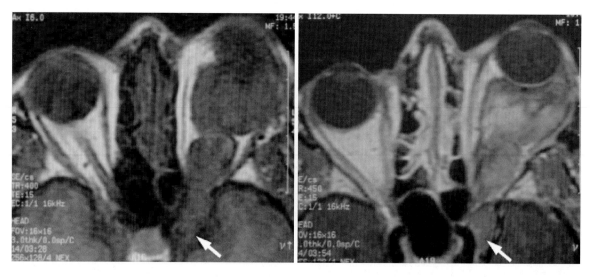

Fig. 4.11. Neurofibroma. Unenhanced T1W (*left*) and enhance T1W (*right*) MR images showing extension of a neurofibroma into the cavernous sinus (*arrows*) along the expected course of cranial nerve V1, helping differentiate it from an optic nerve sheath meningioma which would course along the cranial nerve II

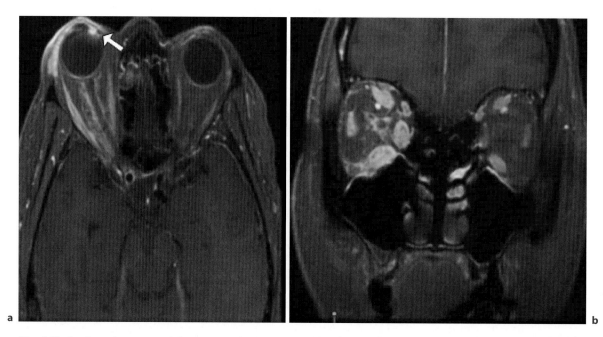

Fig. 4.12a,b. Sarcoidosis. **a** Axial fat suppressed enhanced T1W. **b** Coronal enhanced FS T1W MR images. There is diffuse thickening and enhancement of right optic nerve sheath. Note the granuloma involving the ciliary body (*arrow*) and involvement of the right extra ocular muscles as well

tendency to present with thickening of the dura and leptomeninges (WEBER et al. 1996). Optic nerve sheath sarcoidosis (Fig. 4.12). Lymphoma (Fig. 4.13) and pseudotumor can also be mistaken on imaging for optic nerve sheath meningioma. Optic neuritis may also be mistaken on CT and MRI for optic nerve sheath meningioma. In general, in patients with optic neuritis, contrast enhancement on CT and MR imaging is often

subtle or present in a short segment of the optic nerve, particularly the intracanalicular portion of it. However, at times there may be diffuse unilateral or bilateral optic nerve enhancement mimicking optic nerve sheath meningioma (Fig. 4.14). An *en plaque* meningioma adjacent to the lesser wing of sphenoid can extend into the optic canal, simulating an intracanalicular optic nerve sheath meningioma (Fig. 4.10) (CHARBEL et al. 1999).

4.5.1
Optic Nerve Glioma

Like optic nerve sheath meningioma, MR imaging remains the imaging study of choice for the diagnosis of optic nerve glioma. The tumor may be solitary (Fig. 4.15) or a component of neurofibromatosis-1 (NF-1). Bilateral optic nerve gliomas are characteristic of NF-1 (CHARBEL et al. 1999). In fact, there is a strong association between optic nerve sheath meningiomas and NF-2 that parallels the well-known association of optic nerve gliomas with NF-1 (BOSCH et al. 2006). The

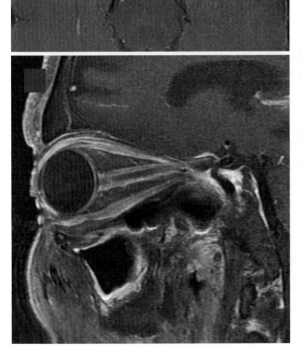

Fig. 4.13. Lymphoma of the optic nerve on 3T magnet. Axial enhanced T1W (*top*) and sagittal enhanced fat suppression T1W (*bottom*) MR images show normal enhancement of the left optic nerve (*arrow*) and marked enhancement around the abnormal right optic nerve sheath. Biopsy of the right optic nerve showed lymphomatoid infiltration of the nerve

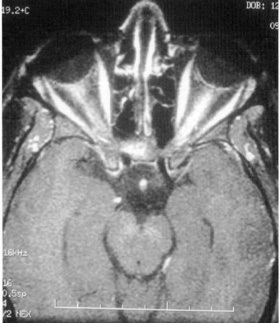

Fig. 4.14. Bilateral optic neuritis in a patient with rheumatoid arthritis. Axial enhanced fat suppressed T1W MR image shows diffuse enhancement of the optic nerves bilaterally

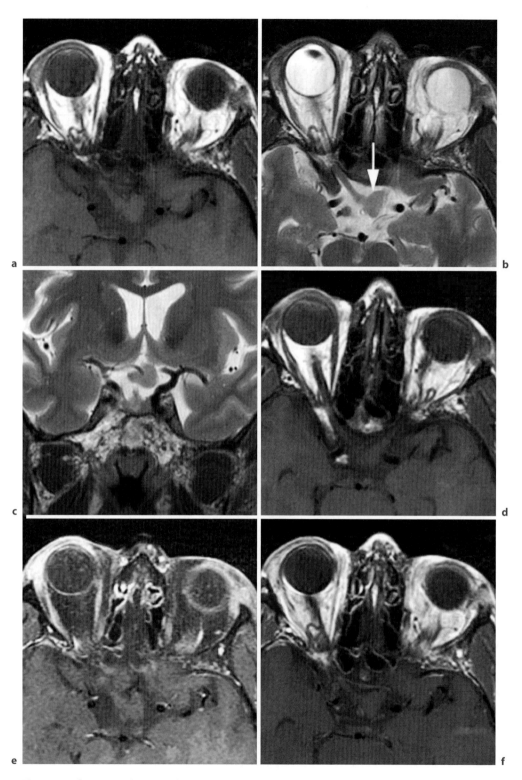

Fig. 4.15a–f. Low grade optic glioma on 3T magnet. **a** Axial T1W. **b** Axial T2W. **c** Coronal T2W. **d** Axial T1W. **e** Axial enhanced fat suppressed T1W. **f** Axial enhanced T1W MR images all showing a presumed optic glioma involving the left optic nerve. (From: Mafee MF, Rapoport M, Karimi A, Ansari S, Shah J (2005) Orbital and ocular imaging using 3- and 1.5-T MR imaging systems. Neuroimag Clin N Am 15:7; with permission)

CT and MRI appearance of optic nerve glioma is often characteristic. The tumor results in marked enlargement along with kinking and buckling of the involved optic nerve (Fig. 4.16, Fig. 4.17). Unlike optic nerve sheath meningioma, cystic changes are commonly seen in optic nerve glioma. At times an optic nerve glioma may not be differentiated on imaging from optic nerve sheath meningioma.

4.6
Miscellaneous

In most cases, the CT and MRI appearance for optic nerve sheath meningioma is quite characteristic. However, at times other rare tumors, such as optic nerve hemangioblastoma, medulloepthelioma, or leptomeningeal carcinomatosis may be mistaken for optic nerve sheath meningiomas. Similarly, a multitude of other orbital tumors can be mistaken for optic nerve sheath meningiomas (Table 4.1), including neurofibroma, schwannoma, fibrous histiocytoma, fibrocytoma, hemangiopericytoma, cavernous hemangioma, lymphangioma, orbital varix, and isolated retrobulbar/optic nerve metastasis (MAFEE et al. 1987; CARMODY et al. 1994). Orbital soft tissue chondrosarcoma is another rare lesion that due to its tendency for tumoral calcification can sometime be mistaken for optic nerve sheath meningioma (Fig. 4.18a,b) (SHINAVER et al. 1997).

On MR imaging, abnormal contrast enhancement of the optic nerve disk and a short segment of the optic nerve just behind the globe has been described in patients with optic neuropathy as a result of cat scratch disease (SCHMALFUSS et al. 2005). Short-segment retrobulbar involvement, however, may be seen in multiple sclerosis, sarcoidosis, and other causes of optic neuropathy (MAFEE 2005b). When short-segment optic nerve sheath enhancement is discovered on MR imaging, we recommend obtaining unenhanced CT images through the orbit with 1.5 mm thickness for the detection of micro/macro-calcification. None of these conditions mentioned above will demonstrate calcification on CT scanning.

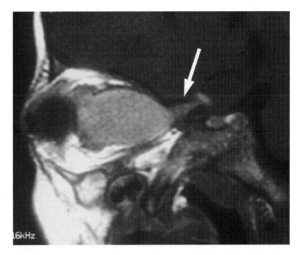

Fig. 4.16. Juvenile pilocytic optic nerve glioma. Sagittal enhanced T1W MR image in a 17-month-old female shows a large mass with intracranial extension to involve the intracranial segment of the optic nerve

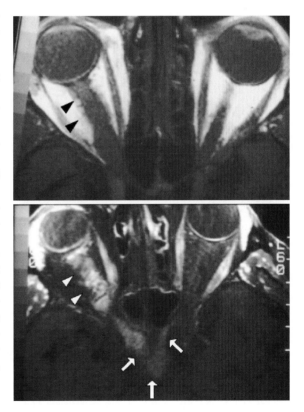

Fig. 4.17. Glioblastoma multiforme of the optic nerve. Unenhanced T1W (*top*) and enhanced T1W with fat saturation (*bottom*) MR images showing irregular thickening of the right optic nerve (*arrowheads*). Note diffuse enhancement extending intra-cranially to involve the intraorbital segment of the contralateral nerve (*arrows*). (Courtesy of A. Flanders, MD, Philadelphia, PA)

Table 4.1. Tumors mimicking optic nerve sheath meningioma

Glioma
Neurofibroma
Schwannoma
Fibrous histiocytoma
Fibrocytoma
Hemangiopericytoma
Cavernous hemangioma
Lymphoma
Lymphangioma
Hemangioblastoma
Medulloepthelioma
Leptomeningeal carcinomatosis
Chondrosarcoma
Solitary retrobulbar/optic nerve metastasis
Orbital varix

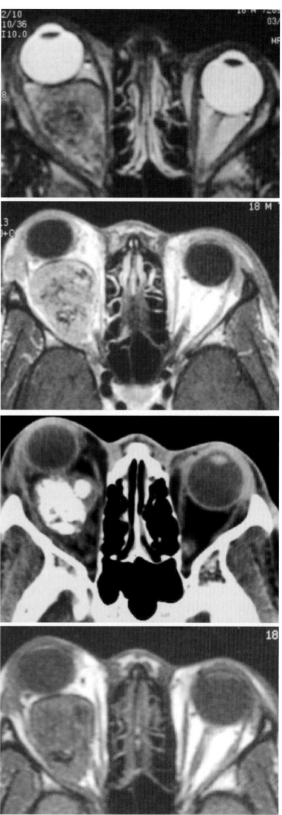

Fig. 4.18. a Orbital mesenchymal chondrosarcoma. T2W (*top*) and enhanced T1W FS (*bottom*) MR images show a large heterogeneously enhancing right retrobulbar mass which surrounds the optic nerve. **b** Orbital mesenchymal chondrosarcoma. Axial unenhanced CT image (*top*) and axial unenhanced T1W MR image in the same patient from Fig. 4.18A showing large mass with coarse calcifications readily identified on the CT image

References

Bosch MM, Wichmann WW, Boltshauser E, Landau K (2006) Optic nerve sheath meningiomas in patients with neurofibromatosis type 2. Arch Ophthalmol Mar 124(3):379–385

Carmody RF, Mafee MF, Goodwin JA et al. (1994) Orbital and optic pathway sarcoidosis: MR findings. AJNR 15:773–783

Charbel FT, Hyun H, Mirsa M et al. (1999) Jaxtaorbital en plaque meningiomas. Report of four cases and review of literature. Radiol Clin North Am 25:89–100

Eddleman CS, Liu JK (2007) Optic nerve sheath meningiomas: current diagnosis and treatment. Neurosurg Focus 23(5):E4

Fox AJ, Debrun G, Vinuela F, Assis L, Coates R (1979) Intrathecal metrizamide cisternography enhancement of optic nerve sheath. J Comput Assist Tomogr 3(5):653–656

Greenberg HS (1998) Meningiomas. In: Gilman S, Goldstein GW, Waxman G (eds) Neurobase. Arbor Publishing, San Diego

Hirst LW, Miller NR, Hodges FJ III, Corbett JJ, Thomspson S (1982) Sphenoid pneumosinus dilatans. A sign of meningioma originating in the optic canal. Neuroradiology 22(4):207–210

Hollander MD, Fitzpatrick, O'Connor SG et al. (1999) Optic gliomas: Radiol Clin North Am 25:59–73

Jacobiec FA, Depot MJ, Kennerdell JS et al. (1984) Combined and computed tomographic diagnostic of orbital glioma and meningioma. Opthamology 91:137

Lee AG, Siebert KJ, Sanan A (1997) Radiologic – clinical correlation: Junctional visual fields loss. AJNR 18:1171

Lloyd GA (1982) Primary orbital meningioma: a review of 41 patients investigated radiologically. Clin Radiol 33:181

Mafee MF (1992) Case 25: optic nerve sheath meningioma. In: Siegel BA, Prato Av (eds) Head and neck disorders (4th series). Test and syllabus. American College of Radiology, Reston, VA, p 533

Mafee MF (1996a) Neuroradiologic imaging of the orbit and globe. In: Bosniak S (ed) Opthalmic plastic and reconstructive surgery. WB Saunders, Philadelphia, p 885

Mafee MF (1996b) Orbital and intraocular lesions. In: Edelman RR, Hesselink JR, Zlatkin MB (eds) Clinical magnetic resonance imaging. WB Saunders, Philadelphia, p 985

Mafee MF. (2005a) The eye and orbit. In: Mafee MF, Valvassori GE, Becker M (eds) Imaging of the head and neck, 2nd edn. Thieme, Stuttgart, Germany, pp 137–294

Mafee MF (2005b) Ocular manifestations of cat-scratch disease: role of MR imaging (editorials). AJNR 26:1303–1304

Mafee MF, Putterman A, Valvarsar GI et al. (1987) Orbital space occupying lesions: role of computed tomography and magnetic resonance imaging. An analysis of 145 cases. Radiol Clin North Am 25:529–559

Mafee MF, Dorodi S, Pai E (1999a) Sarcoidosis of the eye, orbit, and central nervous system. Role of MR imaging. Radiol Clin North Am 25:73–87

Mafee, MF, Goodwin J, Dorodi S (1999b) Optic nerve sheath meningiomas: role of MR imaging. Radiol Clin North Am 25:37–58

Mafee MF, Rapport M, Karimi A et al. (2005) Orbital and ocular imaging using 3- and 1-5 T MR imaging systems. Neuroimaging Clin North Am 15:1–21

Miller NR (2006) New concepts in the diagnosis of management of optic nerve sheath meningioma. J Neuroophthalmol 26(3):200–208

Mouton S, Tilikete C, Bernard M, Krolak-Salmon P, Vighetto A (2007) Optic nerve sheath meningioma: experience in Lyon in twenty patients. Rev Neurol (Paris) 163(5):549–559

Schmalfuss IM, Dean CW, Sistronm C, Bhatti MT (2005) Optic neuropathy secondary to cat-scratch disease: distinguishing MR imaging features from other types of optic neuropathies. AJNR 26:1296–1302

Shinaver CN, Mafee MF, Choi KH (1997) MRI of mesenchymal chondrosarcoma of the orbit; case repor and review of the literature. Neuroradiology 39:296–301

Snell RS, Lamp MA (eds) (1989) Clinical anatomy of the eye. Blackwell Scientific, Boston

Turbin RE, Pokorny K (2004) Diagnosis and treatment of orbital optic nerve sheath meningioma. Cancer Control 11(5):334–341

Walsh FB (1975) Meningiomas primary within the orbit and optic canal. In: Glaser JS, Smith JL (eds) Neuro-opthamology: Symposium of the University of Miami and the Bascom Eye Institute. CV Mosby, St. Louis, p 166

Weber AL, Kwfas R, Pless M (1996) Imaging evaluation of the optic nerve and visual pathway including cranial nerves affecting the visual pathway. Neuroimaging Clin North Am 6:143

Histology and Molecular Genetics

MARKUS J. RIEMENSCHNEIDER and GUIDO REIFENBERGER

CONTENTS

M. J. RIEMENSCHNEIDER, MD
Department of Neuropathology, Heinrich-Heine-University,
Moorenstr. 5, 40225 Duesseldorf, Germany

G. REIFENBERGER, MD, PhD
Department of Neuropathology, Heinrich-Heine-University,
Moorenstr. 5, 40225 Duesseldorf, Germany

KEY POINTS

Optic nerve sheath meningiomas (ONSM) are rare tumors of the anterior visual pathway constituting approximately 2% of all intraorbital tumors and about 1%–2% of meningiomas. They arise from the meningeal coverings of the central nervous system either as primary or secondary orbital lesions. Primary ONSM develop intraorbitally at any location along the optical nerve. They share the same histological features as meningiomas in other locations of the central nervous system and are histologically classified according to the 'World Health Organization (WHO) Classification of Tumours of the Central Nervous System'. Most commonly presenting with a slow growth and a benign clinical behavior, most meningiomas correspond to WHO grade I. Meningothelial and transitional histological variants are the most frequent subtypes of ONSM. However, rare cases are associated with a higher risk of recurrence and shorter survival times. The WHO classification assigns these lesions to WHO grades II and III. This chapter provides a review on meningioma histology in general and about histopathological aspects of ONSM in particular. Moreover, it shortly outlines the underlying molecular alterations that initiate meningioma growth and promote meningioma progression.

Incidence and Epidemiology

Optic nerve sheath meningiomas account for approximately one third of primary optic nerve tumors and 2% of all orbital tumors (DUTTON 1991; EDDLEMAN and LIU 2007; SAEED et al. 2003; WRIGHT et al. 1980, 1989). Like meningiomas in other locations, they are believed to develop from arachnoidal cap cells, though the precise cell of origin of meningiomas has not yet been definitely proven. Optic nerve sheath meningiomas can arise either directly from the intraorbital meningeal coverings of the optic nerve (so-called "primary" optic nerve sheath meningiomas), or they may extend into the orbita from the intracranial cavity following the path of least resistance (so-called "secondary" optic nerve sheath meningiomas) (DUTTON 1992; EDDLEMAN and LIU 2007; SPENCER 1972). Intracranially, the latter variant may originate from the cavernous sinus, falciform ligament, clinoid or sphenoid wing, pituitary fossa, planum sphenoidale or fronto-parieto-temporal areas. The vast majority of optic nerve sheath meningiomas (about 90%) are secondary and thus share identical histologic and molecular genetic features with other central nervous system meningiomas (TURBIN and POKORNY 2004).

Most meningiomas are slowly growing benign lesions. They are most commonly found in middle-aged and elderly patients with a peak incidence in the sixth and seventh decades of life (LOUIS et al. 2007). For optic nerve sheath meningiomas in particular, a lower mean age of manifestation has been reported (42.5 years in women and 36.1 in men; range 3–80 years) (DUTTON 1992). A clear gender preference of about 3:2 towards female patients can be observed for both intracranial and optic nerve sheath meningiomas. This overrepresentation of women is most likely due to the fact that sex hormones, in particular progesterone, are likely involved in meningioma pathogenesis. In line with these findings, pregnancy may exacerbate the growth of meningiomas (BICKERSTAFF et al. 1958; SMITH et al. 2005). Furthermore, approximately two-thirds of meningiomas express progesterone receptors and one-third estrogen receptors (CLAUS et al. 2008). Loss of progesterone receptor expression, however, is observed in more aggressive meningioma types and qualifies as a negative prognostic factor (CARROLL et al. 1993; HSU et al. 1997).

Unlike in adult optic nerve sheath meningiomas, there is no gender preference in tumors that occur in young patients. These tumors are commonly associated with neurofibromatosis type 2 (NF2), an autosomal dominant disorder caused by germline mutations in the *NF2* gene on the long arm of chromosome 22 (BASER et al. 2003). In addition to schwannomas, in particular bilateral vestibular schwannomas, meningiomas are a hallmark feature of this inherited disease. However, half of the sporadic meningiomas also carry mutations in the *NF2* gene, as discussed below in more detail (HARADA et al. 1996; RUTTLEDGE et al. 1994a). Rare familial cases of meningioma have been reported that were not associated with *NF2*, but occurred in patients

with rare hereditary tumor syndromes such as Cowden, Gorlin, Li-Fraumeni, Turcot, Gardener and von Hippel-Lindau syndrome as well as multiple endocrine neoplasia (MEN) type I (ASGHARIAN et al. 2004; LOUIS et al. 1995; LOUIS and VON DEIMLING 1995). However, case numbers are too low to reliably establish causal connections between any of these rare syndromes and meningioma manifestation.

5.2
Histological Classification

5.2.1
Benign Meningioma, WHO Grade I

Meningiomas are histologically classified according to the 2007 WHO classification of tumors of the central nervous system (LOUIS et al. 2007). This classification employs a three-tiered grading scheme mainly based on histologic parameters, which aims to predict the clinical behaviour and prognosis of meningiomas.

More than 80% of intracranial meningiomas and also the vast majority of optic nerve sheath meningiomas are slowly growing tumors of WHO grade I (Tables 5.1 and 5.2). However, it has to be mentioned that histology data about optic nerve sheath meningiomas are restricted because biopsies are often not obtained. This is due to the fact that non-surgical approaches (e.g. radiotherapy) most likely preserve visual function and in regard to clinical outcome are often regarded as superior to surgical approaches (TURBIN and POKORNY 2004).

When histologically evaluated, optic nerve sheath meningiomas most commonly correspond to either the meningothelial or the transitional meningioma variant (BERMAN and MILLER 2006; CARRASCO and PENNE 2004). Meningothelial meningiomas are composed of uniform, epitheloid tumor cells with fuzzy, ill-defined borders, growing in a syncytial manner (Fig. 5.1a). Eosinophilic nuclear cytoplasmatic protrusions, so-called nuclear pseudoinclusions, are another characteristic feature. In addition to meningothelial tumor areas, transitional meningiomas contain spindle-shaped cells resembling fibroblasts that form intersecting facsicles and are often embedded in a collagen- and reticulin-rich matrix. They are histologically characterized by extensive whorl formation, wherein tumor cells wrap around each other forming concentric layers (Fig. 5.1b). These whorls bear a tendency to hyalinize and calcify and then are referred to as psammoma bodies. In the case of psammoma bod-

Table 5.1. Overview of the different histological meningioma variants grouped by WHO grade in accordance with the WHO classification of tumors of the central nervous system (LOUIS et al. 2007)

Meningiomas with low risk of recurrence and aggressive growth	
Meningothelial meningioma	WHO grade I
Fibrous (fibroblastic) meningioma	WHO grade I
Transitional (mixed) meningioma	WHO grade I
Psammomatous meningioma	WHO grade I
Angiomatous meningioma	WHO grade I
Microcystic meningioma	WHO grade I
Secretory meningioma	WHO grade I
Lymphoplasmacyte-rich meningioma	WHO grade I
Metaplastic meningioma	WHO grade I
Meningiomas with greater likelihood of recurrence and/or aggressive behavior	
Atypical meningioma	WHO grade II
Clear cell meningioma	WHO grade II
Chordoid meningioma	WHO grade II
Anaplastic (malignant) meningioma	WHO grade III
Rhabdoid meningioma	WHO grade III
Papillary meningioma	WHO grade III
Meningiomas of any type or grade with high proliferation index and/or brain invasion	

Table 5.2. Histological criteria for meningioma grading in accordance with the WHO classification of tumors of the central nervous system (LOUIS et al. 2007)

Benign meningioma (WHO grade I)
• Any histologic variant other than clear cell, chordoid, papillary, or rhabdoid
• Lack of criteria defining atypical and anaplastic meningioma
Atypical meningioma (WHO grade II) (any of three criteria)
• Elevated mitotic index (≥ 4 mitoses/10 high power fields)
• At least three of the following five parameters:
– Increased cellularity
– High nuclear/cytoplasmatic ratio ("small cells")
– Prominent nucleoli
– Uninterrupted patternless or sheet-like growth
– Foci of spontaneous necrosis (i.e., not induced by embolization or radiation)
• Brain invasion
Anaplastic (malignant) meningioma (grade III) (either of two criteria)
• High mitotic index (≥ 20/10 high power fields)
• Frank anaplasia (sarcoma, carcinoma, or melanoma-like histology)

ies dominating the histological appearance, the tumors are designated psammomatous meningiomas. Another common meningioma variant throughout the CNS, but less common amongst optic nerve sheath meningiomas, is the fibrous or fibroblastic variant, which comprises tumors that are solely composed of spindle-shaped fibroblast-like cells growing in a collagen- and reticulin-rich matrix (Fig. 5.1c,d).

A number of additional, less common benign meningioma variants can be distinguished histologically, including angiomatous, microcystic, secretory, lymphoplasmacyte-rich and metaplastic types (Table 5.1). Al-

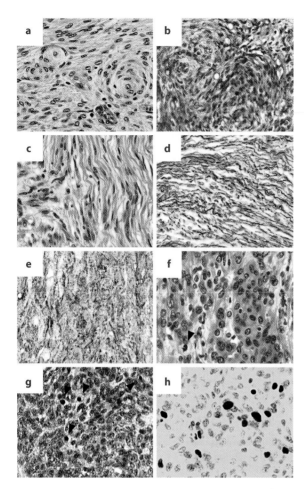

Fig. 5.1a–h. Selected histological features of meningiomas. Most meningiomas are slowly growing tumors of WHO grade I. Note syncytial growth of meningothelial cells in the meningothelial meningioma variant (**a**), formation of multiple meningeal whorls in a transitional meningioma (**b**), and fascicular growth of fibroblast-like spindle cells in the fibrous meningioma variant (**c**). Fibrous meningiomas often contain a dense network of reticulin fibers (**d**). Immunohistochemically, the vast majority of meningiomas stain for epithelial membrane antigen (**e**). Atypical meningiomas of WHO grade II exhibit increased mitotic activity (**f**). Anaplastic meningiomas of WHO grade III are highly cellular tumors with numerous mitoses (**g**) and a high proliferative index as revealed by MIB-1 immunostaining (**h**). *Arrowheads* indicate mitoses (**f, g**). **a,b, c,f,g**: hematoxylin-eosin; **d**: Tibor-Pap silver impregnation; **e**: immunostaining for the epithelial membrane antigen; **h**: immunostaining for the proliferation-associated antigen Ki-67 (clone MIB-1). Original magnification of all images: ×400

beit rare, all these histological variants can potentially be encountered upon microscopic analysis of optic nerve sheath meningiomas, in particular in case of secondary protrusions of primary intracranial tumors into the orbital fossa.

Certain histological variants of meningioma are consistently associated with a more aggressive clinical behavior, in particular chordoid, clear cell, papillary and rhabdoid meningioma variants (Table 5.1). These meningioma subtypes are referred to below.

Optic nerve sheath meningiomas grow along paths of least resistance. Typically, primary lesions remain confined to the subarachnoid or intradural space of the intraorbital optic nerve, secondary tumors arise from the intracranial cavity and grow into this space. However, individual tumors may invade the surrounding dura, orbital tissue, muscle and bone. Also, optic nerve sheath meningiomas tend to grow circumferentially around the optic nerve, thereby interfering with the pial blood supply (CARRASCO and PENNE 2004; KENNERDELL et al. 1988; KIM et al. 2005; WRIGHT et al. 1980,

1989). Although these growth patterns clearly make surgical intervention more difficult and post-operative results less favorable, they are not indicative of atypia or anaplasia. In contrast, invasion of central nervous tissue is associated with higher recurrence and mortality rates similar to atypical meningiomas, even if the tumor appears completely benign otherwise (PERRY et al. 1999).

5.2.2
Atypical Meningioma and Other WHO Grade II Variants

Exact numbers or percentages of atypical meningiomas in the orbital fossa cannot be retrieved from the literature. This may be due to the previously mentioned fact that the diagnosis of optic nerve sheath meningiomas is often solely based on radiographic and clinical findings, while tissue biopsies for histopathological confirmation are not obtained (TURBIN and POKORNY 2004). Nevertheless, as atypical meningiomas make up about

15%–20% of all meningiomas, their histological features may also apply to a subset of optic nerve sheath meningiomas. Atypical meningiomas recur with greater likelihood (about 40% at 5 years) than gross totally resected benign meningiomas (up to 5% at 5 years) (Perry et al. 1997, 1999). As a result, intervals of regular post-surgical clinical follow-up should be shorter in patients with atypical meningiomas.

Histologically, the most important criteria defining atypia is increased mitotic activity, i.e. 4 or more mitoses per 10 microscopic high power fields (Fig. 5.1f). However, in addition to increased mitotic count, the WHO classification also warrants the diagnosis of atypical meningioma if at least three of the following five criteria can be observed: increased cellularity, high nuclear/cytoplasmic ratio ("small cells"), prominent nucleoli, uninterrupted patternless or sheet-like growth, and foci of spontaneous (non-embolization induced) necrosis (Table 5.2).

Brain-invasive, histologically benign and histologically atypical meningiomas both have recurrence and mortality rates similar to those of atypical meningiomas in general (Louis et al. 2007). As such, they should prognostically be considered as WHO grade II lesions.

In addition to the atypical meningiomas classified by the criteria for atypia as described above, certain histological meningioma variants are per se associated with higher recurrence rates and thus graded as WHO grade II (Table 5.1). Chordoid meningiomas typically arise supratentorially and share histological features with chordomas. Characteristically, they are defined by small epithelioid tumor cells containing an eosinophilic or vacuolated cytoplasm (resembling so-called physaliferous cells in chordomas), embedded in a basophilic mucin-rich matrix (Couce et al. 2000). Clear cell meningiomas are composed of sheets of polygonal cells with clear, glycogen-rich, PAS-positive cytoplasm and dense perivascular and interstitial collagen deposition. As clear cell meningiomas typically occur in the posterior fossa and in the spinal cord, this variant seems to be of minor importance in regard to optic nerve sheath meningioma histology (Zorludemir et al. 1995).

5.2.3
Anaplastic (Malignant) Meningioma and Other WHO Grade III Variants

Rare cases of meningiomas (about 1%–3%) can widely infiltrate surrounding tissues and even form remote metastatic deposits (Louis et al. 2007). Thus, these meningiomas meet all criteria applying to other malignant neoplasms. Recurrence rates exceed the ones observed in atypical meningiomas, reaching up to 50%–80%. Median post-surgical survival time is only around 2–3 years (Perry et al. 1999). Histologically, the best defined criterion for anaplasia is mitotic count of 20 or more mitoses per 10 microscopic high power fields (Fig. 5.1g, Table 5.2). Commonly, large zones of geographic necrosis are encountered. However, it is self-explanatory that only spontaneous necroses and not necroses induced by therapeutic embolization have grading implications (Paulus et al. 1993). Some highly malignant meningiomas may be difficult to recognize as primary meningeal neoplasms but may rather resemble sarcoma, carcinoma or melanoma. In rare instances, meningiomas may be so dedifferentiated that the differential diagnostic issue can only be resolved by immunohistochemistry, electron microscopy, or genetic studies.

As for atypical meningiomas, certain meningioma variants are consistently associated with clinically malignant gliomas and therefore classified as WHO grade III tumors (Table 5.1). Papillary meningiomas histologically have a perivascular pseudopapillary growth pattern and can form pseudorosette-like structures similar to those in ependymomas. They often occur in children with high rates of brain invasion, recurrence and metastasis (75%, 55% and 20%, respectively) (Ludwin et al. 1975; Pasquier et al. 1986). Rhabdoid meningiomas contain rounded cells with abundant eosinophilic cytoplasm, eccentrically located nuclei and paranuclear ultrastructural inclusions corresponding to whorled bundles of intermediate filaments (Kepes et al. 1998; Perry et al. 1998a). Both histological variants may manifest as a progression-associated phenotype at the time of recurrence.

5.2.4
Immunohistochemistry

While most benign meningiomas can be easily identified by means of conventional histology, immunohistochemistry may play an important role as a supplement to estimate a tumor's growth activity. The so-called proliferative index is commonly determined with the antibody MIB-1 targeting the Ki-67 antigen (Fig. 5.1h). Ki-67 is a human cell-cycle-related antigen (a nuclear non-histone protein) expressed solely by cycling cells. An elevated proliferative index in meningiomas correlates with an increased risk of recurrence. Despite the fact that counting techniques and cut-off levels are not precisely defined, and staining techniques bear a considerable degree of interlaboratory variability, MIB-1 labeling indices of above 5% are usually considered as being associated with a greater likelihood of recurrence. Thus immunohistochemistry, especially in borderline atypical lesions, may provide additional prognostic information to complement conventional histology (NAKASU et al. 2001; PERRY et al. 1998b). In addition to the expression of the Ki-67 antigen, expression of the progesterone receptor is known to be inversely associated with meningioma grade. Its role in meningioma diagnostics, however, is less well established and its relevance in regard to grading is rather limited (CARROLL et al. 1993; HSU et al. 1997; PERRY et al. 2000).

A second domain of immunohistochemistry in meningioma diagnostics concerns cases that histologically are suspicious of meningioma but lack typical features of meningothelial differentiation. As mentioned above, such tumors may resemble dedifferentiated high-grade lesions or may comprise meningioma variants in which unusual histologic features dominate the histological appearance. Epithelial membrane antigen (EMA, Fig. 5.1e) is the marker most commonly employed in meningioma diagnostics (SCHNITT and VOGEL 1986). In addition, vimentin is strongly expressed in meningiomas (ARTLICH and SCHMIDT 1990). Depending on the differential diagnostic context, staining for these two markers often facilitates the diagnosis. However, both epitopes are not meningioma-specific and the identification of additional meningothelial markers would be highly desirable. In this respect, desmosomal proteins, such as desmoplakin, plakophilin 2, desmocollin 2 and desmoglein 2 have been reported as useful immuno-histochemical markers for meningiomas (AKAT et al. 2003). In addition, claudin 1 has been suggested as a meningioma-associated protein that may be helpful for differential diagnosis (RAJARAM et al. 2004). Secretory meningiomas show a characteristic coexpression of cytokeratins and carcinoembryonic antigen (CEA) in pseudoepithelial tumor cells surrounding pseudopsammoma bodies, while expression of protein S100 may be variably seen in different meningioma subtypes.

5.3
Meningioma Genetics

Studies specifically addressing chromosomal and genetic changes in optic nerve sheath meningiomas are not available due to the rarity of these tumors and the often limited amounts of tumor tissue available for research purposes. Nevertheless, meningiomas in general were among the first solid tumors for which specific chromosomal changes were identified – now more than 40 years ago (ZANG and SINGER 1967; ZANKL and ZANG 1972). Since then, numerous studies have addressed the chromosomal and genetic alterations associated with meningioma development and progression (Table 5.3), which are briefly summarized in the following paragraphs.

Table 5.3. Genetic alterations associated with meningioma initiation and progression. The most common genetic events leading to meningioma initiation comprise losses on chromosome 22q, *NF2* mutations as well as alterations of other members of the protein 4.1 superfamily, such as 4.1B, 4.1R and TSLC1. A plethora of chromosomal copy number changes and alterations of different genetic pathways are involved in the progression from benign to atypical and anaplastic meningioma. The changes summarized in the table are discussed in the text in further detail

Benign meningioma (WHO grade I)	Loss of 22q, *NF2* mutations 4.1B, 4.1R, TSLC1 loss of expression EGFR/PDGFRB activation
Atypical meningioma (WHO grade II)	Losses of 1p, 6q, 10, 14q and 18q gains of 1q, 9q, 12q, 15q, 17q and 20q Notch, WNT, IGF pathway activation progesterone receptor loss of expression telomerase/hTERT activation
Anaplastic meningioma (WHO grade III)	More frequent losses of 6q, 10 and 14q *NDRG2* hypermethylation loss of 9p (*CDKN2A/B, p14*[ARF] homozygous deletion) gain or amplification on 17q23 (*PS6K*, others)

5.3.1
Chromosome 22q, the NF2 Gene and the Protein 4.1 Superfamily

Monosomy 22 is the most frequent chromosomal alteration in meningiomas (Zang 2001). Allelic deletions on chromosome 22 most commonly target the region 22q12.2 harboring the neurofibromatosis 2 (NF2) gene (Dumanski et al. 1987; Seizinger et al. 1987). NF2 is mutated in about 50% of sporadic meningiomas and in all meningiomas that manifest in neurofibromatosis type 2 patients, thus representing the most commonly altered tumor suppressor gene in meningioma pathogenesis (Harada et al. 1996; Leone et al. 1999; Merel et al. 1995; Ruttledge et al. 1994b). More recent studies also report on epigenetic mechanisms contributing to the inactivation of NF2 in menigiomas (Lomas et al. 2005). NF2 mutation or hypermethylation leads to reduced expression of the NF2 gene product merlin, a protein 4.1 superfamily member (Gusella et al. 1999; Rouleau et al. 1993; Trofatter et al. 1993). Functionally, 4.1 proteins serve as linkage molecules between the cell membrane and the cytoskeleton. Merlin localizes to the cell membrane at regions involved in mediating cell-cell contact and regulating cell motility. Merlin binding partners include cell surface proteins, such as CD44 or integrins, and proteins involved in cell cytoskeleton dynamics, like ßII-spectrin, paxillin, actin, and syntenin (James et al. 2001; Jannatipour et al. 2001; Morrison et al. 2001; Obremski et al. 1998; Scoles et al. 1998; Xu and Gutmann 1998). Also, molecules mediating ion transport, such as the sodium hydrogen exchange regulatory factor (NHE-RF), and endocytosis, like the hepatocyte growth factor-regulated tyrosine kinase substrate (HRS), have been proposed as merlin binding partners (Gutmann et al. 2001; Murthy et al. 1998). The functional significance of the individual interrelationships with respect to meningioma pathogenesis are still enigmatic. Nevertheless, it could be demonstrated that binding of CD44 to merlin negatively affects cell proliferation and motility (Shaw et al. 2001; Sherman and Gutmann 2001; Xiao et al. 2002) and that the association between merlin and paxillin seems particularly important for localizing merlin to its appropriate subcellular location (Fernandez-Valle et al. 2002).

In addition to merlin, certain other protein 4.1 family members have been shown to play a role in meningioma biology. Protein 4.1B, the gene product of the DAL-1 gene, is commonly downregulated in meningiomas, particularly in higher grade cases, and executes its tumor suppressor function via Rac1-dependent c-Jun-NH2-kinase signaling (Gerber et al. 2006; Gutmann et al. 2000; Nunes et al. 2005). Protein 4.1 R is also frequently inactivated in sporadic meningiomas and – when active – inhibits meningioma cell growth (Robb et al. 2003).

While on chromosome 22q NF2 is by far the most important tumor suppressor gene in meningiomas, the frequency of deletions in this chromosomal region exceeds that of NF2 mutations and in rare meningioma cases also deletions outside the NF2 region have been described (Lomas et al. 2002). These results encouraged the search for tumor suppressor genes other than NF2 on chromosome 22q in meningiomas, but yielded only a few additional candidates, such as the MN1, the INI1 and the BAM22 genes. In a series of 126 meningiomas, 3% of the tumors bore an identical exon 9 mutation in INI1 (Schmitz et al. 2001). No BAM22 mutations were identified in 110 meningiomas, despite downregulation of BAM22 transcripts in 13% of cases (Peyrard et al. 1994, 1996). MN1 at 22q12.1 was reported to be lost in a patient with multiple meningiomas who had an intact NF2 gene; however, gene function is that of a transcription factor rather than a tumor suppressor (Lekanne Deprez et al. 1995). Finally, the LARGE gene at 22q12.3 has been proposed as another promising candidate, but due to its size this gene has not yet undergone mutational analysis (Peyrard et al. 1999).

5.3.2
Progression-associated Genetic Changes

Loss of chromosome 22q and NF2 mutation most commonly manifest at the stage of benign meningiomas and do not relevantly increase in frequency with malignant progression. Thus, these molecular alterations are early events in meningiomagenesis and may be of relevance to meningioma initiation, in particular in fibrous and transitional meningioma variants. The molecular changes conveying progression from benign to atypical (WHO grade II) and anaplastic (WHO grade III) meningioma are complex and numerous (Table 5.3). Cytogenetically, atypical meningiomas show frequent losses on chromosomes 1p, 6q, 10, 14q, 18q and gains on 1q, 9q, 12q, 15q, 17q and 20q. Anaplastic meningiomas have more frequent losses on 6q, 10 and 14q, additional losses on 9p, and gains or amplifications on 17q23 (Buschges et al. 2002; Lamszus et al. 1999; Ozaki et al. 1999; Weber et al. 1997).

Loss of chromosome 1p is the second most common cytogenetic aberration in meningiomas and the most common progression-associated genomic alteration. The following genes have been suggested as candidate tumor suppressor genes on 1p in meningiomas: TP73, CDKN2C (encoding p18[INK4c]), RAD54L and ALPL

(Bostrom et al. 2001; Lomas et al. 2001; Mendiola et al. 1999; Niedermayer et al. 1997). However, none of these genes exhibited mutations consistently or frequently enough to indicate clearly its role as the major candidate tumor suppressor in meningiomas; their promoter methylation status, as a means of epigenetic inactivation, has not yet been assessed in a comprehensive manner. Interestingly, recent studies identified multiple promoter-associated CpG islands in meningiomas with 1p loss, and promoter hypermethylation of the *TP73* was identified in 13 out of 30 meningiomas with 1p deletions (Bello et al. 2004; Lomas et al. 2004).

Several putative target genes located in other regions of frequent chromosomal gains and losses in meningiomas have been studied for abnormalities. For example, the *PTEN* gene on 10q23 has been studied extensively, but homozygous deletions were absent and mutations restricted to rare cases of meningiomas (Peters et al. 1998). Similarly, alterations of the *TP53* gene at 17p13 are uncommon in meningiomas, though allelic losses on 17p are observed in a subset of higher-grade lesions (Bostrom et al. 2001; Wang et al. 1995). Few chromosomal aberrations could be clearly linked to specific genes. These include the common loss of chromosome arm 9p, which targets the tumor suppressor genes *CDKN2A* (encoding $p16^{INK4a}$), *p14*^{ARF} and *CDKN2B* (encoding $p15^{INK4b}$) at 9p21 (Bostrom et al. 2001; Ruas and Peters 1998). Functionally, dysregulation of $p16^{INK4a}$, $p14^{ARF}$ and $p15^{INK4b}$ disturbs pRB- and p53-cell cycle regulation (Prives and Hall 1999). About 70% of anaplastic meningiomas carry 9p21 deletions, with the corresponding patients showing significantly shorter survival as compared to patients with anaplastic meningiomas lacking this alteration (Perry et al. 2002). The *NDRG2* gene maps to the long arm of chromosome 14 and is often transcriptionally down-regulated by promoter hypermethylation in anaplastic meningiomas and clinically aggressive atypical meningiomas (Lusis et al. 2005). Other authors reported on gain and/or amplification of the ribosomal protein S6 kinase gene (*PS6K*) in a minor fraction of anaplastic meningiomas, suggesting a role for *PS6K* in meningioma progression (Buschges et al. 2002; Cai et al. 2001). However, other genes located close to *PS6K* at 17q23-q24 may also be targets of amplification in anaplastic meningiomas (Buschges et al. 2002; Cai et al. 2001).

Another recently identified mechanism promoting meningioma progression is telomerase activation. Telomerase is an enzymatic complex that is specifically involved in maintaining telomeres, the very ends of linear chromosomes (Kalala et al. 2005; Leuraud et al. 2004). While activation of the reverse transcription subunit hTERT (reverse telomerase transcriptase) was re-

stricted to 37% of benign meningiomas, it was detected in nearly all WHO grade II and III tumors (up to 95%), and correlated with a higher risk of recurrence, malignancy and shorter progression free survival (Maes et al. 2005; Simon et al. 2001).

With respect to novel means of targeted therapy, it has to be mentioned that molecular aberrations in meningiomas have been linked to the disturbance of certain well-defined signaling pathways, which in turn might be targeted by specific antibodies or small molecules (Table 5.3). For example, activation of the growth factor receptors EGFR (epidermal growth factor receptor) and PDGFRB (platelet-derived growth factor receptor ß) commonly occurs in benign meningiomas and thus represents an early alteration involved in meningioma initiation (Carroll et al. 1997; Johnson et al. 1994; Jones et al. 1990; Shamah et al. 1997; Weisman et al. 1987). In contrast, changes in the pRB- and p53-cell cycle regulation pathways as well as activation of Notch, WNT and IGF signaling appear to be linked to more invasive and aggressive meningioma phenotypes (Bostrom et al. 2001; Cuevas et al. 2005; Wrobel et al. 2005).

The application of modern methods for large-scale genomic and expression profiling of meningiomas has revealed several additional novel aspects. For example, a recent study challenged the conventional three-tiered grading system for meningiomas by providing molecular evidence that expression profiles in atypical meningiomas are similar to either benign or malignant meningiomas, thus suggesting a subdivision of meningiomas into only two main molecular groups designated as 'low-proliferative' and 'high-proliferative' meningiomas (Carvalho et al. 2007). Yet other studies suggested that distinct mRNA expression profiles are associated with spinal versus intracranial meningiomas (Sayagues et al. 2006), meningiomas from male versus female patients (Tabernero et al. 2007), as well as progesterone-positive versus -negative meningiomas (Claus et al. 2008). However, since optic nerve sheath meningiomas have not been subjected to any systematic genetic or expression profiling, it remains unclear whether these particular tumors are associated with any specific molecular signature that distinguishes them from meningiomas in other locations.

References

Akat K, Mennel HD, Kremer P, Gassler N, Bleck CK, Kartenbeck J (2003) Molecular characterization of desmosomes in meningiomas and arachnoidal tissue. Acta Neuropathol 106:337–347

Artlich A. Schmidt D (1990) Immunohistochemical profile of meningiomas and their histological subtypes. Hum Pathol 21:843–849

Asgharian B, Chen YJ, Patronas NJ, Peghini PL, Reynolds JC, Vortmeyer A, Zhuang Z, Venzon DJ, Gibril F, Jensen RT (2004) Meningiomas may be a component tumor of multiple endocrine neoplasia type 1. Clin Cancer Res 10:869–880

Baser ME, Evans GR, Gutmann DH (2003) Neurofibromatosis 2. Curr Opin Neurol 16:27–33

Bello MJ, Aminoso C, Lopez-Marin I, Arjona D, Gonzalez-Gomez P, Alonso ME, Lomas J, de Campos JM, Kusak ME, Vaquero J, Isla A, Gutierrez M, Sarasa JL, Rey JA (2004) DNA methylation of multiple promoter-associated CpG islands in meningiomas: relationship with the allelic status at 1p and 22q. Acta Neuropathol (Berl) 108:413–421

Berman D, Miller NR (2006) New concepts in the management of optic nerve sheath meningiomas. Ann Acad Med Singapore 35:168–174

Bickerstaff ER, Small JM, Guest IA (1958) The relapsing course of certain meningiomas in relation to pregnancy and menstruation. J Neurol Neurosurg Psychiatry 21:89–91

Bostrom J, Meyer-Puttlitz B, Wolter M, Blaschke B, Weber RG, Lichter P, Ichimura K, Collins VP, Reifenberger G (2001) Alterations of the tumor suppressor genes CDKN2A (p16(INK4a)), p14(ARF), CDKN2B (p15(INK4b)), and CDKN2C (p18(INK4c)) in atypical and anaplastic meningiomas. Am J Pathol 159:661–669

Buschges R, Ichimura K, Weber RG, Reifenberger G, Collins VP (2002) Allelic gain and amplification on the long arm of chromosome 17 in anaplastic meningiomas. Brain Pathol 12:145–153

Cai DX, James CD, Scheithauer BW, Couch FJ, Perry A (2001) PS6K amplification characterizes a small subset of anaplastic meningiomas. Am J Clin Pathol 115:213–218

Carrasco JR, Penne RB (2004) Optic nerve sheath meningiomas and advanced treatment options. Curr Opin Ophthalmol 15:406–410

Carroll RS, Glowacka D, Dashner K, Black PM (1993) Progesterone receptor expression in meningiomas. Cancer Res 53:1312–1316

Carroll RS, Black PM, Zhang J, Kirsch M, Percec I, Lau N, Guha A (1997) Expression and activation of epidermal growth factor receptors in meningiomas. J Neurosurg 87:315–323

Carvalho LH, Smirnov I, Baia GS, Modrusan Z, Smith JS, Jun P, Costello JF, McDermott MW, Vandenberg SR, Lal A (2007) Molecular signatures define two main classes of meningiomas. Mol Cancer 6:64

Claus EB, Park PJ, Carroll R, Chan J, Black PM (2008) Specific genes expressed in association with progesterone receptors in meningioma. Cancer Res 68:314–322

Couce ME, Aker FV, Scheithauer BW (2000) Chordoid meningioma: a clinicopathologic study of 42 cases. Am J Surg Pathol 24:899–905

Cuevas IC, Slocum AL, Jun P, Costello JF, Bollen AW, Riggins GJ, McDermott MW, Lal A (2005) Meningioma transcript profiles reveal deregulated Notch signaling pathway. Cancer Res 65:5070–5075

Dumanski JP, Carlbom E, Collins VP, Nordenskjold M (1987) Deletion mapping of a locus on human chromosome 22 involved in the oncogenesis of meningioma. Proc Natl Acad Sci U S A 84:9275–9279

Dutton JJ (1991) Optic nerve gliomas and meningiomas. Neurol Clin 9:163–177

Dutton JJ (1992) Optic nerve sheath meningiomas. Surv Ophthalmol 37:167–183

Eddleman CS, Liu JK (2007) Optic nerve sheath meningioma: current diagnosis and treatment. Neurosurg Focus 23:E4

Fernandez-Valle C, Tang Y, Ricard J, Rodenas-Ruano A, Taylor A, Hackler E, Biggerstaff J, Iacovelli J (2002) Paxillin binds schwannomin and regulates its density-dependent localization and effect on cell morphology. Nat Genet 31:354–362

Gerber MA, Bahr SM, Gutmann DH (2006) Protein 4.1B/differentially expressed in adenocarcinoma of the lung-1 functions as a growth suppressor in meningioma cells by activating Rac1-dependent c-Jun-NH(2)-kinase signaling. Cancer Res 66:5295–5303

Gusella JF, Ramesh V, MacCollin M, Jacoby LB (1999) Merlin: the neurofibromatosis 2 tumor suppressor. Biochim Biophys Acta 1423:M29–36

Gutmann DH, Donahoe J, Perry A, Lemke N, Gorse K, Kittiniyom K, Rempel SA, Gutierrez JA, Newsham IF (2000) Loss of DAL-1, a protein 4.1-related tumor suppressor, is an important early event in the pathogenesis of meningiomas. Hum Mol Genet 9:1495–1500

Gutmann DH, Haipek CA, Burke SP, Sun CX, Scoles DR, Pulst SM (2001) The NF2 interactor, hepatocyte growth factor-regulated tyrosine kinase substrate (HRS), associates with merlin in the "open" conformation and suppresses cell growth and motility. Hum Mol Genet 10:825–834

Harada T, Irving RM, Xuereb JH, Barton DE, Hardy DG, Moffat DA, Maher ER (1996) Molecular genetic investigation of the neurofibromatosis type 2 tumor suppressor gene in sporadic meningioma. J Neurosurg 84:847–851

Hsu DW, Efird JT, Hedley-Whyte ET (1997) Progesterone and estrogen receptors in meningiomas: prognostic considerations. J Neurosurg 86:113–120

James MF, Manchanda N, Gonzalez-Agosti C, Hartwig JH, Ramesh V (2001) The neurofibromatosis 2 protein product merlin selectively binds F-actin but not G-actin, and stabilizes the filaments through a lateral association. Biochem J 356:377–386

Jannatipour M, Dion P, Khan S, Jindal H, Fan X, Laganiere J, Chishti AH, Rouleau GA (2001) Schwannomin isoform-1 interacts with syntenin via PDZ domains. J Biol Chem 276:33093–33100

Johnson MD, Horiba M, Winnier AR, Arteaga CL (1994) The epidermal growth factor receptor is associated with phospholipase C-gamma 1 in meningiomas. Hum Pathol 25:146–153

Jones NR, Rossi ML, Gregoriou M, Hughes JT (1990) Epidermal growth factor receptor expression in 72 meningiomas. Cancer 66:152–155

Kalala JP, Maes L, Vandenbroecke C, de Ridder L (2005) The hTERT protein as a marker for malignancy in meningiomas. Oncol Rep 13:273–277

Kennerdell JS, Maroon JC, Malton M, Warren FA (1988) The management of optic nerve sheath meningiomas. Am J Ophthalmol 106:450–457

Kepes JJ, Moral LA, Wilkinson SB, Abdullah A, Llena JF (1998) Rhabdoid transformation of tumor cells in meningiomas: a histologic indication of increased proliferative activity: report of four cases. Am J Surg Pathol 22:231–238

Kim JW, Rizzo JF, Lessell S (2005) Controversies in the management of optic nerve sheath meningiomas. Int Ophthalmol Clin 45:15–23

Lamszus K, Kluwe L, Matschke J, Meissner H, Laas R, Westphal M (1999) Allelic losses at 1p, 9q, 10q, 14q, and 22q in the progression of aggressive meningiomas and undifferentiated meningeal sarcomas. Cancer Genet Cytogenet 110:103–110

Lekanne Deprez RH, Riegman PH, Groen NA, Warringa UL, van Biezen NA, Molijn AC, Bootsma D, de Jong PJ, Menon AG, Kley NA et al. (1995) Cloning and characterization of MN1, a gene from chromosome 22q11, which is disrupted by a balanced translocation in a meningioma. Oncogene 10:1521–1528

Leone PE, Bello MJ, de Campos JM, Vaquero J, Sarasa JL, Pestana A, Rey JA (1999) NF2 gene mutations and allelic status of 1p, 14q and 22q in sporadic meningiomas. Oncogene 18:2231–2239

Leuraud P, Dezamis E, Aguirre-Cruz L, Taillibert S, Lejeune J, Robin E, Mokhtari K, Boch AL, Cornu P, Delattre JY, Sanson M (2004) Prognostic value of allelic losses and telomerase activity in meningiomas. J Neurosurg 100:303–309

Lomas J, Bello MJ, Arjona D, Gonzalez-Gomez P, Alonso ME, de Campos JM, Vaquero J, Ruiz-Barnes P, Sarasa JL, Casartelli C, Rey JA (2001) Analysis of p73 gene in meningiomas with deletion at 1p. Cancer Genet Cytogenet 129:88–91

Lomas J, Bello MJ, Alonso ME, Gonzalez-Gomez P, Arjona D, Kusak ME, de Campos JM, Sarasa JL, Rey JA (2002) Loss of chromosome 22 and absence of NF2 gene mutation in a case of multiple meningiomas. Hum Pathol 33:375–378

Lomas J, Aminoso C, Gonzalez-Gomez P, Eva Alonso M, Arjona D, Lopez-Marin I, de Campos JM, Isla A, Vaquero J, Gutierrez M, Sarasa JL, Josefa Bello M, Rey JA (2004) Methylation status of TP73 in meningiomas. Cancer Genet Cytogenet 148:148–151

Lomas J, Bello MJ, Arjona D, Alonso ME, Martinez-Glez V, Lopez-Marin I, Aminoso C, de Campos JM, Isla A, Vaquero J, Rey JA (2005) Genetic and epigenetic alteration of the NF2 gene in sporadic meningiomas. Genes Chromosomes Cancer 42:314–319

Louis DN, von Deimling A (1995) Hereditary tumor syndromes of the nervous system: overview and rare syndromes. Brain Pathol 5:145–151

Louis DN, Ramesh V, Gusella JF (1995) Neuropathology and molecular genetics of neurofibromatosis 2 and related tumors. Brain Pathol 5:163–172

Louis DN, Ohgaki H, Wiestler OD, Cavenee WK (eds) (2007) WHO classification of tumours of the central nervous system, 3rd edn. IARC Press, Lyon

Ludwin SK, Rubinstein LJ, Russell DS (1975) Papillary meningioma: a malignant variant of meningioma. Cancer 36:1363–1373

Lusis EA, Watson MA, Chicoine MR, Lyman M, Roerig P, Reifenberger G, Gutmann DH, Perry A (2005) Integrative genomic analysis identifies NDRG2 as a candidate tumor suppressor gene frequently inactivated in clinically aggressive meningioma. Cancer Res 65:7121–7126

Maes L, Lippens E, Kalala JP, de Ridder L (2005) The hTERT-protein and Ki-67 labelling index in recurrent and nonrecurrent meningiomas. Cell Prolif 38:3–12

Mendiola M, Bello MJ, Alonso J, Leone PE, Vaquero J, Sarasa JL, Kusak ME, De Campos JM, Pestana A, Rey JA (1999) Search for mutations of the hRAD54 gene in sporadic meningiomas with deletion at 1p32. Mol Carcinog 24:300–304

Merel P, Hoang-Xuan K, Sanson M, Moreau-Aubry A, Bijlsma EK, Lazaro C, Moisan JP, Resche F, Nishisho I, Estivill X et al. (1995) Predominant occurrence of somatic mutations of the NF2 gene in meningiomas and schwannomas. Genes Chromosomes Cancer 13:211–216

Morrison H, Sherman LS, Legg J, Banine F, Isacke C, Haipek CA, Gutmann DH, Ponta H, Herrlich P (2001) The NF2 tumor suppressor gene product, merlin, mediates contact inhibition of growth through interactions with CD44. Genes Dev 15:968–980

Murthy A, Gonzalez-Agosti C, Cordero E, Pinney D, Candia C, Solomon F, Gusella J, Ramesh V (1998) NHE-RF, a regulatory cofactor for Na(+)-H+ exchange, is a common interactor for merlin and ERM (MERM) proteins. J Biol Chem 273:1273–1276

Nakasu S, Li DH, Okabe H, Nakajima M, Matsuda M (2001) Significance of MIB-1 staining indices in meningiomas: comparison of two counting methods. Am J Surg Pathol 25:472–478

Niedermayer I, Feiden W, Henn W, Steilen-Gimbel H, Steudel WI, Zang KD (1997) Loss of alkaline phosphatase activity in meningiomas: a rapid histochemical technique indicating progression-associated deletion of a putative tumor suppressor gene on the distal part of the short arm of chromosome 1. J Neuropathol Exp Neurol 56:879–886

Nunes F, Shen Y, Niida Y, Beauchamp R, Stemmer-Rachamimov AO, Ramesh V, Gusella J, MacCollin M (2005) Inactivation patterns of NF2 and DAL-1/4.1B (EPB41L3) in sporadic meningioma. Cancer Genet Cytogenet 162:135–139

Obremski VJ, Hall AM, Fernandez-Valle C (1998) Merlin, the neurofibromatosis type 2 gene product, and beta1 integrin associate in isolated and differentiating Schwann cells. J Neurobiol 37:487–501

Ozaki S, Nishizaki T, Ito H, Sasaki K (1999) Comparative genomic hybridization analysis of genetic alterations associated with malignant progression of meningioma. J Neurooncol 41:167–174

Pasquier B, Gasnier F, Pasquier D, Keddari E, Morens A, Couderc P (1986) Papillary meningioma. Clinicopathologic study of seven cases and review of the literature. Cancer 58:299–305

Paulus W, Meixensberger J, Hofmann E, Roggendorf W (1993) Effect of embolisation of meningioma on Ki-67 proliferation index. J Clin Pathol 46:876–877

Perry A, Stafford SL, Scheithauer BW, Suman VJ, Lohse CM (1997) Meningioma grading: an analysis of histologic parameters. Am J Surg Pathol 21:1455–1465

Perry A, Scheithauer BW, Stafford SL, Abell-Aleff PC, Meyer FB (1998a) "Rhabdoid" meningioma: an aggressive variant. Am J Surg Pathol 22:1482–1490

Perry A, Stafford SL, Scheithauer BW, Suman VJ, Lohse CM (1998b) The prognostic significance of MIB-1, p53, and DNA flow cytometry in completely resected primary meningiomas. Cancer 82:2262–2269

Perry A, Scheithauer BW, Stafford SL, Lohse CM, Wollan PC (1999) "Malignancy" in meningiomas: a clinicopathologic study of 116 patients, with grading implications. Cancer 85:2046–2056

Perry A, Cai DX, Scheithauer BW, Swanson PE, Lohse CM, Newsham IF, Weaver A, Gutmann DH (2000) Merlin, DAL-1, and progesterone receptor expression in clinicopathologic subsets of meningioma: a correlative immunohistochemical study of 175 cases. J Neuropathol Exp Neurol 59:872–879

Perry A, Banerjee R, Lohse CM, Kleinschmidt-DeMasters BK, Scheithauer BW (2002) A role for chromosome 9p21 deletions in the malignant progression of meningiomas and the prognosis of anaplastic meningiomas. Brain Pathol 12:183–190

Peters N, Wellenreuther R, Rollbrocker B, Hayashi Y, Meyer-Puttlitz B, Duerr EM, Lenartz D, Marsh DJ, Schramm J, Wiestler OD, Parsons R, Eng C, von Deimling A (1998) Analysis of the PTEN gene in human meningiomas. Neuropathol Appl Neurobiol 24:3–8

Peyrard M, Fransson I, Xie YG, Han FY, Ruttledge MH, Swahn S, Collins JE, Dunham I, Collins VP, Dumanski JP (1994) Characterization of a new member of the human beta-adaptin gene family from chromosome 22q12, a candidate meningioma gene. Hum Mol Genet 3:1393–1399

Peyrard M, Pan HQ, Kedra D, Fransson I, Swahn S, Hartman K, Clifton SW, Roe BA, Dumanski JP (1996) Structure of the promoter and genomic organization of the human beta'-adaptin gene (BAM22) from chromosome 22q12. Genomics 36:112–117

Peyrard M, Seroussi E, Sandberg-Nordqvist AC, Xie YG, Han FY, Fransson I, Collins J, Dunham I, Kost-Alimova M, Imreh S, Dumanski JP (1999) The human LARGE gene from 22q12.3-q13.1 is a new, distinct member of the glycosyltransferase gene family. Proc Natl Acad Sci U S A 96:598–603

Prives C, Hall PA (1999) The p53 pathway. J Pathol 187:112–126

Rajaram V, Brat DJ, Perry A (2004) Anaplastic meningioma versus meningeal hemangiopericytoma: immunohistochemical and genetic markers. Hum Pathol 35:1413–1418

Robb VA, Li W, Gascard P, Perry A, Mohandas N, Gutmann DH (2003) Identification of a third Protein 4.1 tumor suppressor, Protein 4.1R, in meningioma pathogenesis. Neurobiol Dis 13:191–202

Rouleau GA, Merel P, Lutchman M, Sanson M, Zucman J, Marineau C, Hoang-Xuan K, Demczuk S, Desmaze C, Plougastel B et al. (1993) Alteration in a new gene encoding a putative membrane-organizing protein causes neurofibromatosis type 2. Nature 363:515–521

Ruas M, Peters G (1998) The p16INK4a/CDKN2A tumor suppressor and its relatives. Biochim Biophys Acta 1378:F115–177

Ruttledge MH, Sarrazin J, Rangaratnam S, Phelan CM, Twist E, Merel P, Delattre O, Thomas G, Nordenskjold M, Collins VP et al. (1994a) Evidence for the complete inactivation of the NF2 gene in the majority of sporadic meningiomas. Nat Genet 6:180–184

Ruttledge MH, Xie YG, Han FY, Peyrard M, Collins VP, Nordenskjold M, Dumanski JP (1994b) Deletions on chromosome 22 in sporadic meningioma. Genes Chromosomes Cancer 10:122–130

Saeed P, Rootman J, Nugent RA, White VA, Mackenzie IR, Koornneef L (2003) Optic nerve sheath meningiomas. Ophthalmology 110:2019–2030

Sayagues JM, Tabernero MD, Maillo A, Trelles O, Espinosa AB, Sarasquete ME, Merino M, Rasillo A, Vera JF, Santos-Briz A, de Alava E, Garcia-Macias MC, Orfao A (2006) Microarray-based analysis of spinal versus intracranial meningiomas: different clinical, biological, and genetic characteristics associated with distinct patterns of gene expression. J Neuropathol Exp Neurol 65:445–454

Schmitz U, Mueller W, Weber M, Sevenet N, Delattre O, von Deimling A (2001) INI1 mutations in meningiomas at a potential hotspot in exon 9. Br J Cancer 84:199–201

Schnitt SJ, Vogel H (1986) Meningiomas. Diagnostic value of immunoperoxidase staining for epithelial membrane antigen. Am J Surg Pathol 10:640–649

Scoles DR, Huynh DP, Morcos PA, Coulsell ER, Robinson NG, Tamanoi F, Pulst SM (1998) Neurofibromatosis 2 tumour suppressor schwannomin interacts with betaII-spectrin. Nat Genet 18:354–359

Seizinger BR, de la Monte S, Atkins L, Gusella JF, Martuza RL (1987) Molecular genetic approach to human meningioma: loss of genes on chromosome 22. Proc Natl Acad Sci U S A 84:5419–5423

Shamah SM, Alberta JA, Giannobile WV, Guha A, Kwon YK, Carroll RS, Black PM, Stiles CD (1997) Detection of activated platelet-derived growth factor receptors in human meningioma. Cancer Res 57:4141–4147

Shaw RJ, Paez JG, Curto M, Yaktine A, Pruitt WM, Saotome I, O'Bryan JP, Gupta V, Ratner N, Der CJ, Jacks T, Mc-Clatchey AI (2001) The Nf2 tumor suppressor, merlin, functions in Rac-dependent signaling. Dev Cell 1:63–72

Sherman LS, Gutmann DH (2001) Merlin: hanging tumor suppression on the Rac. Trends Cell Biol 11:442–444

Simon M, Park TW, Koster G, Mahlberg R, Hackenbroch M, Bostrom J, Loning T, Schramm J (2001) Alterations of INK4a(p16-p14ARF)/INK4b(p15) expression and telomerase activation in meningioma progression. J Neurooncol 55:149–158

Smith JS, Quinones-Hinojosa A, Harmon-Smith M, Bollen AW, McDermott MW (2005) Sex steroid and growth factor profile of a meningioma associated with pregnancy. Can J Neurol Sci 32:122–127

Spencer WH (1972) Primary neoplasms of the optic nerve and its sheaths: clinical features and current concepts of pathogenetic mechanisms. Trans Am Ophthalmol Soc 70:490–528

Tabernero MD, Espinosa AB, Maillo A, Rebelo O, Vera JF, Sayagues JM, Merino M, Diaz P, Sousa P, Orfao A (2007) Patient gender is associated with distinct patterns of chromosomal abnormalities and sex chromosome linked gene-expression profiles in meningiomas. Oncologist 12:1225–1236

Trofatter JA, MacCollin MM, Rutter JL, Murrell JR, Duyao MP, Parry DM, Eldridge R, Kley N, Menon AG, Pulaski K et al. (1993) A novel moesin-, ezrin-, radixin-like gene is a candidate for the neurofibromatosis 2 tumor suppressor. Cell 72:791–800

Turbin RE, Pokorny K (2004) Diagnosis and treatment of orbital optic nerve sheath meningioma. Cancer Control 11:334–341

Wang JL, Zhang ZJ, Hartman M, Smits A, Westermark B, Muhr C, Nister M (1995) Detection of TP53 gene mutation in human meningiomas: a study using immunohistochemistry, polymerase chain reaction/single-strand conformation polymorphism and DNA sequencing techniques on paraffin-embedded samples. Int J Cancer 64:223–228

Weber RG, Bostrom J, Wolter M, Baudis M, Collins VP, Reifenberger G, Lichter P (1997) Analysis of genomic alterations in benign, atypical, and anaplastic meningiomas: toward a genetic model of meningioma progression. Proc Natl Acad Sci U S A 94:14719–14724

Weisman AS, Raguet SS, Kelly PA (1987) Characterization of the epidermal growth factor receptor in human meningioma. Cancer Res 47:2172–2176

Wright JE, Call NB, Liaricos S (1980) Primary optic nerve meningioma. Br J Ophthalmol 64:553–558

Wright JE, McNab AA, McDonald WI (1989) Primary optic nerve sheath meningioma. Br J Ophthalmol 73:960–966

Wrobel G, Roerig P, Kokocinski F, Neben K, Hahn M, Reifenberger G, Lichter P (2005) Microarray-based gene expression profiling of benign, atypical and anaplastic meningiomas identifies novel genes associated with meningioma progression. Int J Cancer 114:249–256

Xiao GH, Beeser A, Chernoff J, Testa JR (2002) p21-activated kinase links Rac/Cdc42 signaling to merlin. J Biol Chem 277:883–886

Xu HM, Gutmann DH (1998) Merlin differentially associates with the microtubule and actin cytoskeleton. J Neurosci Res 51:403–415

Zang KD (2001) Meningioma: a cytogenetic model of a complex benign human tumor, including data on 394 karyotyped cases. Cytogenet Cell Genet 93:207–220

Zang KD, Singer H (1967) Chromosomal consitution of meningiomas. Nature 216:84–85

Zankl H, Zang KD (1972) Cytological and cytogenetical studies on brain tumors. 4. Identification of the missing G chromosome in human meningiomas as no. 22 by fluorescence technique. Humangenetik 14:167–169

Zorludemir S, Scheithauer BW, Hirose T, Van Houten C, Miller G, Meyer FB (1995) Clear cell meningioma. A clinicopathologic study of a potentially aggressive variant of meningioma. Am J Surg Pathol 19:493–505

Surgery in Primary Optic Nerve Sheath Meningioma

Roger E. Turbin and John S. Kennerdell

CONTENTS

KEY POINTS

Various surgical procedures, depending on the extent of the tumor, have been practiced in patients with primary optic nerve sheath meningioma. Extirpation, sometimes including removal of the optic nerve from chiasm to globe, have occasionally been suggested. Some have proposed microsurgical resection, but patients risk high probability of postoperative blindness due to almost certain inadvertent dissection of the pial vasculature. Despite cases with isolated surgical benefit, the long-term experience of surgical manipulation of ONSM is limited. Several articles addressing intra-cranial meningioma undergoing gross total resection have indicated that residual tumor remains in situ and may even be spread during surgery. Therefore, surgical resection alone will not result in cure of "focal" tumors, and partial nerve sheath surgery could result in orbital recurrence. Although transient postoperative improvement is well documented after relief of congestion, it is typically of brief duration. Extirpative surgery is rarely required and obviously associated with complete and irreversible loss of function as well as potential for significant other morbidity and mortality. Therefore, radiation therapy most likely still represents the best treatment option for long-term preservation of vision in ONSM patients with progressive visual loss.

R. E. Turbin, MD, FACS
Assistant Professor, Neuro-ophthalmology and Orbital Surgery, University of Medicine and Dentistry, New Jersey Medical School (UMDNJ-NJMS), 90 Bergen Street, Suite 6177, Newark, NJ 07103, USA

J. S. Kennerdell, MD
Chairman and Professor Emeritus, Allegheny General Hospital, 320 East North Ave, Suite 116, Pittsburgh, PA 15212, USA

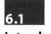

Introduction

The management of optic nerve sheath meningioma (ONSM) has undergone evolution over the last few decades. Observation, followed by surgical extirpation when disfiguring proptosis, intracranial extension, or severe visual loss occurred, was considered by some to be the standard of care (Dutton 1992; Wright et al. 1989; Alper 1981; Egan and Lessell 2002). Others have described a more aggressive approach based on age, suggesting complete extirpation of the optic nerve from chiasm to globe in all patients under age 30 despite the presence of relatively preserved vision (Wright et al. 1989). Some authors have been proponents of microsurgical resection, but patients risk high probability of postoperative blindness due to almost certain inadvertent dissection of the pial vasculature (Dutton 1992; Rosenberg and Miller 1984). Several other reports have also discussed the potential benefits of surgical intervention for ONSM in specific clinical scenarios including focal anterior tumors, cases of constrictive tumors causing congestive optic disc swelling, and canalicular compressive lesions (Watson and Greenwood 1968; Ebers et al. 1980; Alper 1981; Smith et al. 1981; Guyer et al. 1985; Ito et al. 1988; Kennerdell et al. 1988; Clark et al. 1989; Cristante 1994; Saeed et al. 2003; Schick et al. 2004; Turbin et al. 2006; Jaggi et al. 2007).

Treatment Goals

Short, intermediate, and long term stabilization of visual function remain the established primary treatment goal of ONSM. Secondary goals include recovery of recently acquired visual deficits and local control of tumor growth. Achievement of these primary and secondary goals occasionally must be considered independently due to a number of factors subsequently discussed. Furthermore, the establishment of stabilization of visual function as a primary goal of therapy, though seemingly "a priori", has only relatively recently become accepted as a feasible goal in a majority of patients (Turbin et al. 2002; Dutton 1992; Wright et al. 1989; Alper 1981; Egan and Lessell 2002; Miller 2002).

Some patients with primary ONSM have nonprogressive disease, while others present for the first time during active phases of growth or visual loss. A subgroup develop growth or visual loss many years into

periods of long-term clinical stability. Finally, others develop radiographic or clinical growth without visual decline or visual decline without documented growth. These concepts have contributed to historical controversy in the management of these infrequent tumors, and remain important guides when assessing risk benefit ratios of treatment paradigms. That being said, most patients with primary ONSM develop progressive visual dysfunction leading to ipsilateral blindness over years (Turbin et al. 2002).

Factors that affect the likelihood for successful stabilization of visual function are incompletely understood but may be related to intrinsic tumor cell activity and turnover, proliferative indices, ultra structure of tumor, as well as extent and location of tumor mass. Yet most treatment decisions remain based on clinical and radiographic assessments, without histologic confirmation of tumor. Therefore, the decision to treat typically is based primarily on documented clinical or occasionally radiographic progression. Divided dose, conformal radiotherapy remains to date the primary treatment modality most likely to obtain the primary and secondary treatment goals listed above, although selection of optimal treatment strategy remains an active topic of study (Andrews et al. 2002; Becker et al. 2002; Liu et al. 2002; Narayan et al. 2003; Pitz et al. 2002; Turbin et al. 2002; Saeed et al. 2003; Baumert et al. 2003; Richards et al. 2005).

A Subset of Data on Surgery in Primary ONSM

We recently reviewed our results of long-term visual outcome in patients with primary ONSM, a subset of whom underwent either surgery or surgery in combination with irradiation (Turbin et al. 2002). A total of 64 patients were identified with a mean follow up period of 150.2 months (range 51–516, SD 74.7). Patients with follow-up of shorter than 50 months were excluded. For the 59 patients used in statistical analysis, the mean follow-up was 138.5 months (range 57–277, SD 55.4). The diagnosis was confirmed by histopathologic examination in 32 cases. Of the 64 patients, 5 were excluded from statistical analysis because of the NLP vision criteria.

6.3.1
Demographics

Of 59 patients with vision greater than NLP at diagnosis, 13 were observed only, 12 had surgery only (4 bi-

Table 6.1. Surgical description of 33 patients undergoing surgical biopsy, subtotal or total resection[a]

Operation	Number	Description
Needle biopsy (or ONSF[†])	8	Four required additional surgical intervention (one ONSF[†], two orbitotomy, one craniotomy)
Orbitotomy (subtotal or total)	9	Two required additional craniotomy, one required embolization and craniotomy[‡]
Craniotomy (subtotal or total)	16	Four required additional surgical intervention three craniotomy, one ONSF[†]

*Five patients treated with at least one surgical intervention were excluded due to the no light perception criteria (1 needle biopsy, 1 orbitotomy, and 2 cranitoy).
[†]Optic nerve sheath decompression for persistent nerve head edema.
[‡]See case presented in text.
ONSF - optic nerve sheath fenestration; NLP - no light perception

[a]From Table 4, Turbin RE, Thompson CR, Kennerdell JS et al. (2002) A long-term visual outcome comparison in patients with optic nerve sheath meningioma managed with observation, surgery, or surgery and radiotherapy. Ophthalmology 109:890–899

opsy or partial resection, 8 total resection), 18 received radiation alone, 16 had surgery and radiation (14 biopsy or partial resection and radiation, 2 patients total resection and radiation). Of the five patients who were NLP at diagnosis, one had a partial resection, and four had total resection. Of the eight patients who underwent needle biopsy or optic nerve sheath fenestration, four had additional surgical procedures. Of the nine patients undergoing subtotal or total resection by orbitotomy, three required further surgical procedures. Of the 16 patients who underwent subtotal or total excision by craniotomy (which may have included orbitotomy as well), 4 required additional surgical procedures (Table 6.1).

6.3.2
Results

Four patients who were observed, seven patients who had surgery alone, and eight patients who had surgery and radiation developed radiographic progression. No patient developed subsequent spread to the other optic nerve in any group, although six patients had bilateral disease at presentation. When visual acuity at last follow-up was compared with visual acuity at diagnosis for each group, visual acuity fell significantly for the observed only, surgery only and surgery with radiation groups. The radiation only group showed a decrease in visual acuity that was not significant from the baseline. When comparing vision at diagnosis or at treatment to vision at last follow-up, 8 of 18 (44.4%) patients treated with radiation and 5 of 16 (31.3%) patients treated with

surgery followed by radiation, showed at least two lines of improvement (including improvement from light perception to finger counting) that remained stable through the last follow-up.

Only 2 of 25 (8%) patients not treated with radiation ever improved at least one line of Snellen acuity. One patient (previously reported in 1978) with a rare focal "globular" nerve sheath meningioma, had the tumor completely resected, but it recurred in the orbit, although vision was preserved at 20/25 as late as 1997 (Mark et al. 1978). Another patient developed severe worsening of vision during pregnancy, which spontaneously improved post-partum. The tumor ultimately extended intracranially, and was excised in its entirety, leaving NLP vision.

6.3.3
Complications

Patients treated with surgery alone developed a complication related to therapy in 66.7% (two cases of vascular occlusion, two cases neovascular glaucoma, one cerebrospinal fluid leak, two cases of severe ocular motility deficit, one case of neurotrophic exposure). Patients treated with radiation and surgery developed a complication related to therapy in 62.5% of cases (two cases of retinopathy/vascular occlusion, two cases neovascular glaucoma, one cerebral infarct and concurrent cerebrospinal fluid leak, two cases of severe motility deficit, one case of persistent iritis, one case of recurrent orbital hemorrhage, one case of lymphoma). It is difficult to assess if surgical or combination therapy increased the susceptibility to treatment complications, because of varied therapies and surgical approaches.

6.4
General Indications for Surgical Intervention

Diagnosis of primary ONSM is typically based on clinical and radiographic criteria without histologic confirmation. Similarly, vision preserving treatment paradigms are primarily based on various radiotherepeutic options, often without histologic confirmation. However, on occasion atypical clinical or radiographic characteristics lead to sufficient clinical uncertainty to require histologic confirmation of ONSM rather than to rely on an empiric course of corticosteroids to rule out other inflammatory lesions. Therefore biopsy remains a reasonable option in selected cases. In other cases, lesions which are focal, exophytic and predominantly extradural may anatomically lend themselves to near total resection. Surgical extirpation also remains an option if intracranial spread threatens contralateral visual pathways and ipsilateral recovery of visual function is hopeless, or severe proptosis and the ocular surface abnormalities it causes are disfiguring or otherwise unmanageable. Surgery may remain an option in selected patients with a constrictive compartment syndrome of the intraorbital optic nerve causing congestive optic nerve edema with macular edema. Finally, surgery remains a viable option in patients with secondary meningioma of nearby intracranial structures that affect the optic nerve. Each of these clinical indications are subsequently discussed in more detail.

6.4.1
Diagnostic Biopsy

In atypical cases, biopsy remains an important option and is the commonest indication for which I operate on these lesions. Although many lesions that mimic optic nerve sheath meningioma will respond to radiotherapy, some inflammatory lesions require ongoing, lesion specific immunosuppressive therapy. In addition, malignant lesions exist that require systemic staging or other modes of systemic and local control (Fig. 6.1a,b). Biopsy may be performed in a limited fashion via needle aspiration or via transorbital approaches. These techniques have been well described and are beyond the scope of this chapter. The biopsy itself may give temporary improvement in visual function that is probably short lived via decompressive effects (Kennerdell et al. 1988; Cristante 1994; Turbin et al. 2006; Dutton 1992). Recurrence or spread into periorbital tissues may occur (Wright et al. 1989), and the biopsy should usually be followed by radiotherapy after lesion confirmation (Turbin et al. 2006; Saeed et al. 2003).

6.4.1.1
Case (from Turbin et al. 2006)

A 32-year-old woman developed loss of visual acuity over 5 months to 20/300 in the left eye (OS). She had 1 mm of left proptosis, mild resistance to retropulsion, and a 4+ RAPD OS. The funduscopic examination revealed disc edema of the left optic nerve with telangiectasia. A high-resolution MRI showed diffuse enhancement of the intra-orbital left optic nerve sheath complex. The optic nerve substance, rather than the

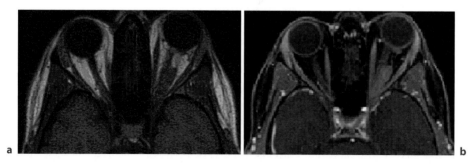

Fig. 6.1a,b. Axial T1 (**a**) and axial T1 fat suppressed with contrast (**b**) orbital MRI of a middle-aged woman with no significant medical problems. Images show a predominantly tubular exophytic lesion lateral to the left optic nerve extending from the orbital apex to mid-orbital optic nerve. Biopsy via orbitotomy revealed malignant lymphoid cells consistent with lymphoma. Courtesy of Mask J Kupersmith, MD

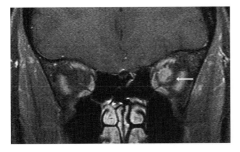

Fig. 6.2. Coronal T1 fat suppressed contrast enhanced MRI show an enlarged optic nerve/sheath complex. In retrospect, the small hypodense nonenhancing signal at the inferior-lateral aspect of the nerve sheath likely represents a compressed optic nerve within enhancing meningioma. This photograph was adapted from an image also used by the American Academy of Ophthalmology: Turbin RE, optic Nerve Sheath Meningioma. American Academy of Ophthalmology Anaheim, CA. November 15, 2003

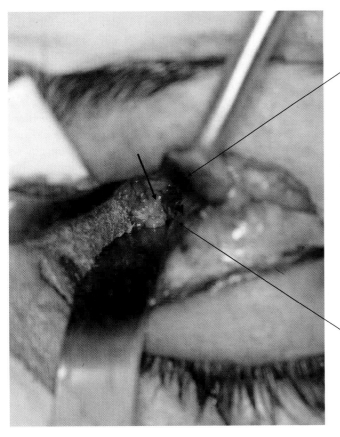

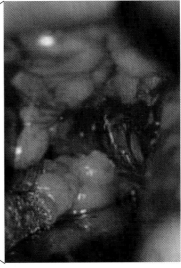

Fig. 6.3. An intraoperative photograph, oriented with the eyebrow *located at the top of the image* and eyelashes of the left upper eyelid *located at the bottom of the image.* The *long arrow* represents the deep orbital fat immediately medial and adjacent to the enlarged optic nerve complex. The *inset* better shows the optic nerve complex, which is visualized as a white structure underneath the pial plexus of posterior ciliary vessels. Courtesy of Roger Turbin, MD

sheath and subarachnoid space, appeared to be radiographically enlarged (Fig 6.2). Intracanalicular and possibly intracranial involvement were present. The patient refused consideration of biopsy and radiation therapy, and the acuity fell to no light perception (NLP) over the next two months despite two courses of intravenous and oral corticosteroid therapy.

Given the rapidly progressive course and unusual appearance of the MRI, the patient underwent a diagnostic left optic nerve sheath biopsy with removal of a large window of dura using a superior-medial lid crease orbitotomy (Fig. 6.3) (Pelton and Patel 2001). Extruding tumor was gently removed in a piecemeal fashion (Fig. 6.4). The pathologic examination confirmed ONSM. In retrospect, subsequent magnified views confirmed the nerve was compressed eccentrically within an abnormal and expanded sheath. The patient elected to undergo subsequent orbital irradiation and was

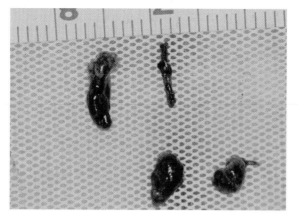

Fig. 6.4. Piecemeal stripping of histopathologically confirmed primary ONSM obtained via superior medial orbitotomy. This component of tumor easily extruded after incising the optic nerve sheath. No attempt to aggressively dissect the tumor was attempted, which would lead to damage to pial vascular architecture. Adapted from Figure 5 of Turbin RE, Wladis EJ, Frohman LP, et al. Role for surgery as adjuvant therapy in optic nerve sheath meningioma. Ophthal Plast Reconstr Surg 2006;22(4):278–82

treated with a five field technique using 3-D conformal radiation therapy with 5040 cGy over 6 weeks (LINAC, 6MEV, stereotactic frame).

The disc edema improved immediately postoperatively and her acuity began to improve prior to beginning her radiotherapy. Six and a half years later, her visual field and acuity (20/200) remain stable, and no orbital tumor spread has occurred.

6.4.2
Decompression of Compartment Syndrome

Although radiation therapy remains the vision-preserving treatment of choice given progressive visual dysfunction, the authors believe that a role may still exist for surgical therapy as an adjuvant to radiation in a very highly selected subset of patients who have otherwise few options. We previously reported the characteristics of two unusual patients experiencing dramatic improvement in vision after nerve sheath surgery with biopsy for ONSM (Turbin et al. 2006) and discussed a potential role and reasonable selection criteria for this intervention. Others have reported both long term (10 years) and short lived effects (2 years) of this intervention (Saeed et al. 2003; Wright 1977)

We believe that these cases support the hypothesis that nerve sheath surgery may provide a useful adjuvant therapy to radiotherapy in highly selected cases with significant nerve head congestion, optic nerve compres-

sion, fulminant visual loss, and few treatment options. These patients represent a very highly selected subset and we have utilized this management only twice for this role, although other patients in our's and other's series have shown improvement after limited resection. Ideally, radiotherapy should be utilized prior to the development of rapid visual loss. However, in cases with orbital ONSM meeting these criteria, it may be possible to improve visual outcome by decompressing the optic nerve. The procedure should consist of the surgical approach most likely to generate a wide view of the involved segment of the nerve based on radiographic images (medial orbitotomy, lateral orbitotomy with bone flap, or superior-medial eyelid crease orbitotomy). A wide dural window should be removed, followed by excision of extruding mass. If the tumor does not extrude, the surgeon should confirm that the nerve substance itself is not expanded, and gently tease the superficial surface of the mass to obtain the biopsy, while avoiding visible vessels. However, more aggressive attempts at removal of tumor are rarely indicated. Bleeding at the operative site may be controlled with a fibrous absorbable hemostatic agent, which we typically remove at the end of the case. Patients not previously irradiated should be strongly encouraged to undergo therapy to prevent spread of intraorbital tumor (Turbin et al. 2006).

6.4.2.1
Case

A 39-year-old woman, who initially presented with a 6-year history of ipsilateral gradual progressive optic neuropathy and abduction deficit was treated with 28 sessions of fractionated stereotactic radiation over 37 days (Xknife 3.0, 4MV Ph, stereotactic frame) totaling 5040 cGY. Her visual acuity improved from 20/25 to 20/20 OS, her chronic disc edema resolved, although the optic nerve became pale and choroidal folds persisted. Approximately 2 years later, visual acuity decreased to 20/200 in the left eye (20/20 OD). Her RAPD OS severely worsened and she could not distinguish color plates. Funduscopic exam revealed recurrence of marked disc edema with macular and peripapillary exudates. The disc edema and macular exudates continued to worsen over the next 6 months, but no other findings suggested super-imposed radiation-induced optic neuropathy or retinopathy (Fig. 6.5a). A repeat MRI was unchanged and again showed findings consistent with stable ONSM (Fig. 6.6). Because of the unusual clinical course, the patient underwent a left lateral orbitotomy to biopsy the lesion and decompress the congested optic nerve sheath later that month. At the

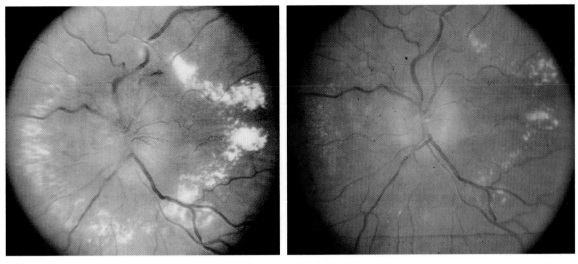

Fig. 6.5. a Preoperative fundus photograph showing severe congestive disc edema and macular exudation approximately 2 years after receiving radiotherapy. Visual acuity dropped to 20/200, and was accompanied by progressive intensity of an ipsilateral afferent pupillary defect. Typical vascular changes of radiation retinopathy were lacking, and the findings were assumed to be related to perioptic congestion from the constrictive orbital meningioma. **b** Significant resolution of optic nerve and macular edema with return of visual acuity to 20/25. Adapted from Figure 1 of Turbin RE, Wladis EJ, Frohman LP, et al. Role for surgery as adjuvant therapy in optic nerve sheath meningioma. Ophthal Plast Reconstr Surg 2006;22(4):278–82

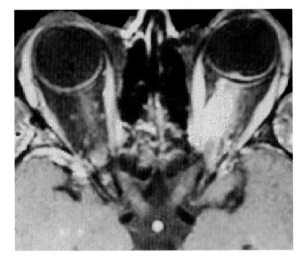

Fig. 6.6. Unchanged radiographic enlargement and extensive enhancement of the left ONSM from the orbital apex to the globe two years after radiotherapy. Adapted from Figure 5 of Turbin RE, Wladis EJ, Frohman LP, et al. Role for surgery as adjuvant therapy in optic nerve sheath meningioma. Ophthal Plast Reconstr Surg 2006;22(4):278–82

time of surgery, an enlarged nerve sheath complex was visualized. The sheath was incised and a dural window was created. Minute fragments of superficial tissue from within the sheath were removed in a piecemeal fashion. Film tumor did not actively extrude, possibly because of changes from previous radiation therapy. However, no attempt was made to remove deep fragments within the sheath. Immediate postoperative visual acuity fell transiently to no light perception OS for approximately twelve hours. A brief course (three doses, 250 mg) of in-travenous postoperative methylprednisolone improved her postoperative vision to 10/400. She was discharged on a rapidly tapering course of 80 mg of prednisone over the following week. The histopathologic evaluation was consistent with meningioma. By postoperative week five, significant postoperative improvement in the exudative disc edema occurred (Fig. 6.5b), and the visual acuity improved to 20/25 OS. The acuity remains 20/25 9 years later, and her visual field remains stable. No orbital spread has occurred at the site of the biopsy.

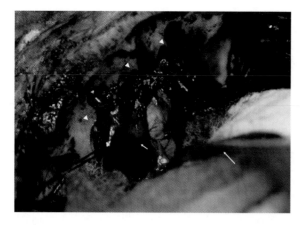

Fig. 6.7. Fronto-temporal craniotomy with unroofing of the left orbit allows for exposure of the intraorbital optic nerve complex. The scalloped, cut edge of the orbital roof is marked by *white arrowheads*, and is located at the *top* of the photograph. The levator superioris is retracted laterally with a traction suture. The superior rectus is marked by a *small white arrow*, and the frontal lobe is retracted underneath the malleable retractor at the *bottom* of the image (*long white arrow*). Courtesy of Paul Langer, MD

6.4.3
Role of Resection

Predominantly extradural, focal nerve sheath lesions or ectopic orbital tumors are very rare but may be resected, leaving a rim of meningeal tissue that does not disrupt pial blood supply. In fact, the most commonly cited case reported by Mark et al. (1978) developed local recurrence (without visual loss), and was re-reported in a later publication (Turbin et al. 2002). Other authors report total excision with improvement of vision and no tumor recurrence (Saeed et al. 2003).

In cases of primary ONSM, patients must be carefully selected, consented for complete visual loss, and approached via transorbital or transcranial extradural orbitotomy to allow microsurgical techniques using the operating microscope.

6.4.4
Resection as Extirpative Surgery

Advances in neuroimaging, greater access to medical care, and greater acceptance of the use of early radiotherapy have resulted in fewer cases of primary ONSM requiring extirpative surgery in developed countries.

Cases with severe proptosis are much less common than in patients with optic nerve glioma, and secondary orbital meningioma. With improved techniques and access to MRI imaging, few cases of ONSM require preventative extirpation. When these cases occur, access to the orbits is obtained via a combined transcranial orbitotomy. With frontal lobe retracted, the orbital roof is resected providing access to the distal optic nerve as it approaches the globe. The intracranial optic nerve is resected proximal to the chiasm, and the nerve-sheath tumor complex is removed en bloc (Fig. 6.7).

6.4.5
Resection of Secondary ONSM

Discussion of this topic is important to contrast primary and secondary ONSM. The clinical similarities and differences of primary and secondary ONSM are important to consider because differences between these two entities emphasize fundamental differences in treatment strategies. These two entities may be difficult to clinically differentiate, present with similar manifestations, and are frequently discussed together by authors. Differences in lesion architecture and especially anatomic location lend support to a greater surgical role in patients with secondary ONSM. The same is not typically true of primary ONSM, nor secondary ONSM that invades the intraorbital nerve sheath or its pial vasculature. Delineation of the surgical goals therefore remain remains an important concept in selecting surgical candidates.

In experienced hands, partial tumor resection is possible with good visual outcome in patients with intracranial meningioma that secondarily affect the optic nerve; this disease remains a surgical entity (Schick et al. 2004). Schick and colleagues developed a classification based on tumor location which emphasizes location of secondary ONSM that may be amenable to partial resection. These authors provide impressive evidence that their group could decompress the intracranial optic canal from a pterional intradural (54 patients) or extradural approach (10 patients) with relative safety and relatively low incidence (21.7%) of iatrogenic visual loss. The authors reported a transient nonvisual morbidity of 12.3% and permanent morbidity of 2.7%, with 5 cases of worsening vision in each of 2 groups of 29 patients with good vision (Snellen >0.5) and 17 with fair vision (Snellen 0.5 to 0.1). Of note, in the groups of fair vision and poor vision, four patients and two patients had improvement of vision (15.4%) from the surgical procedure.

6.5
Canalicular Involvement

Tumor that involves the intracanalicular segment of the optic nerve remains a more controversial issue and decisions are often considered on a case by case basis and vary regionally. Optic nerve meningioma may also primarily or secondarily affect the canalicular segment of the optic nerve. Some authors have projected the surgical principal of optic canal decompression in secondary meningioma to selected patients with intracanalicular primary ONSM (MILLER 2002; CRISTANTE 1994; YUCEER et al. 1994; VERHEGGEN et al. 1996; JACKSON et al. 2003).

JACKSON et al. (2003) described three patients in a series of six with intracanalicular primary ONSM. Visual data supplied by the authors is limited and confirmatory postoperative images are not provided, but authors describe "vision preserved" in three patients with complete surgical resection of the lesion. CRISTANTE (1994) also described three patients who underwent "an unroofing of the optic canal as well as a longitudinal incision of the optic sheath" approached through a combined extradural and intradural pterional craniotomy. In his series of primary and secondary ONSM, 27 of 68 operations included the unroofing of the optic canal. Cristante concluded, however, based on his and others' observations (AL-MEFTY and SMITH 1991; ANDREWS and WILSON 1988), that invasion of the optic canal in any form lends itself only "rare(ly) to postoperative improvement in visual function."

6.6
Conclusion

Despite these and other cases with isolated surgical benefit, the long-term effect of surgical manipulation of ONSM is not known. Several articles addressing intracranial meningioma undergoing gross total resection have indicated that residual tumor remains in situ and may even be spread during surgery. Therefore, surgical resection alone will not result in cure of "focal" tumors, and partial nerve sheath surgery could result in orbital recurrence. Although transient postoperative improvement is well documented after relief of congestion, it is typically of brief duration. Extirpative surgery is rarely required and obviously associated with complete and irreversible loss of function as well as potential for significant other morbidity and mortality. Therefore, radiation therapy most likely still represents the best treatment option for long-term preservation of vision in ONSM patients with progressive visual loss.

References

Al-Mefty O, Smith RR (1991) Tuberculum sellae meningiomas. In: Al-Mefty O (ed) Meningiomas, Raven, New York, pp 395–411

Alper MG (1981) Management of optic nerve sheath meningiomas. J Clin Neuro-Ophthalmol 1:101–117

Andrews BT, Wilson CB (1998) Suprasellar meningiomas. The effect of tumor location on postoperative visual outcome. J Neurosurg 69:523–528

Andrews DW, Faroozan R, Yang BP et al. (2002) Fractionated stereotactic radiotherapy for the treatment of optic nerve sheath meningiomas: preliminary observations of 33 optic nerves in 30 patients with historical comparison to observation with or without prior surgery. Neurosurg 51:809–904

Baumert BG, Norton IA, Davis JB (2003) Intensity-modulated stereotactic radiotherapy vs. stereotactic conformal radiotherapy for the treatment of meningioma located predominantly in the skull base. Int J Radiat Oncol Biol Phys 57:580–592

Becker G, Jeremic B, Pitz S et al. (2002) Stereotactic fractionated radiotherapy in patients with optic nerve sheath meningioma. Int J Radiat Oncol Biol Phys 54:1422–1429

Clark WC, Theofilos CS, Fleming JC (1989) Primary optic nerve sheath meningiomas. J Neurosurg 70:37–40

Cristante L (1994) Surgical treatment of meningiomas of the orbit and optic canal: a retrospective study with particular attention to the visual outcome. Acta Neurochir 126:27–32

Dutton JJ (1992) Optic nerve sheath meningiomas. Surv Ophthalmol 37:167–183

Ebers GC, Girvin JP, Canny CB (1980) A possible optic nerve meningioma. Arch Neurol 37:781–783

Egan RA, Lessell S (2002) A contribution to the natural history of optic nerve sheath meningiomas. Arch Ophthalmol 120:1505–1508

Guyer DR, Miller NR, Long DM et al. (1985) Visual function following optic canal decompression via craniotomy. J Neurosurg 62:631–638

Ito M, Ishizawa A, Miyaoaka M et al. (1988) Intraorbital meningiomas: surgical management and role of radiation therapy. Surg Neurol 29:448–453

Jackson A, Patankar T, Laitt RD (2003) Intracanalicular optic nerve meningima: a serious diagnostic pitfall. Am J Neuroradiol 24(6):1167–1170

Jaggi JV, Mironov A, Huber AR et al. (2007) Optic nerve compartment syndrome in a patient with optic nerve sheath meningioma. Eur J Ophthalmol 17:454–458

Kennerdell JS, Maroon JC, Malton M et al. (1988) The management of optic nerve sheath meningiomas. Am J Ophthalmol 106:450–457

Liu JK, Forman S, Hershewe GL et al. (2002) Optic nerve sheath meningiomas: visual improvement after stereotactic radiotherapy. Neurosurg 50:950–957

Mark LE, Kennerdell JS, Maroon JC et al. (1978) Microsurgical removal of a primary intraorbital meningioma. Am J Ophthalmol 86:704–709

Miller NR (2002) Radiation for optic nerve meningiomas: is this the answer? Ophthalmology 109:833–834

Narayan S, Cornblath WT, Sandler HM et al. (2003) Preliminary visual outcomes after three-dimensional conformal radiation therapy for optic nerve sheath meningioma. Int J Radiat Oncol Biol Phys 56:537–543

Pelton RW, Patel BC (2001) Superomedial lid crease approach to the medial intraconal space: a new technique for access to the optic nerve and central space. Ophthal Plast Reconstr Surg 17:241–253

Pitz S, Becker G, Schiefer U et al. (2002) Stereotactic fractionated irradiation of optic nerve sheath meningioma: a new treatment alterative. Br J Ophthalmol 86:1265–1268

Richards JC, Roden D, Harper CS (2005) Management of sight-threatening optic nerve sheath meningioma with frationated stereotactic radiotherapy. Clin Experiment Ophthalmol 33(2):137–141

Rosenberg LF, Miller NR (1984) Visual results after microsurgical removal of meningiomas involving the anterior visual system. Arch Ophthalmol 102:1019–1023

Saeed P, Rootman J, Nugent RA et al. (2003) Optic nerve sheath meningiomas. Ophthalmology 110:2019–2030

Schick U, Dott U, Hassler W (2004) Surgical management of meningiomas involving the optic nerve sheath. J Neurosurg 101:951–959

Smith JL, Vuksanovic MM, Yates BM et al. (1981) Radiation therapy for optic nerve meningiomas. J Clin Neuro-Ophthalmol 1:85–99

Turbin RE, Thompson CR, Kennerdell JS et al. (2002) A long-term visual outcome comparison in patients with optic nerve sheath meningioma managed with observation, surgery, or surgery and radiotherapy. Ophthalmology 109:890–899

Turbin RE, Wladis EJ, Frohman LP et al. (2006) Role for surgery as adjuvant therapy in optic nerve sheath meningioma. Ophthal Plast Reconstr Surg 22(4):278–282

Verheggen R, Markakis E, Mühlendyck H et al. (1996) Symptomatology, surgical therapy and postoperative results of sphenoorbital, intraorbital-intracanalicular and optic sheath meningiomas. Acta Neurochir Suppl 65:95–98

Watson AG, Greenwood WR (1968) Meningioma of the optic nerve. Can J Ophthalmol 3(2):181–183

Wright JE (1977) Primary optic nerve meningiomas: clinical presentation and management. Trans AM Acad Ophthalmol 83:617–625

Wright JE, McNab AA, McDonald WI (1989) Primary optic nerve sheath meningioma. Br J Ophthalmol 73:960–966

Yüceer N, Erdogan A, Ziya H (1994) Primary optic nerve sheath meningiomas. Report of seven cases (clinical neuroradiological, pathological and surgical considerations in seven cases). J Neurosurg Sci 38(3):155–159

7

Conventional Radiation Therapy in Primary Optic Nerve Sheath Meningioma

Branislav Jeremić

CONTENTS

KEY POINTS

Conventional RT provided consistently good results in patients with pONSM. However, more recent, 3D conformal and stereotactic RT achievements in this disease showed that the latter two techniques have major advantage over more traditional 2D RT. This is so regarding both tumour control and toxicity. Both issues are superiorly addressed by more sophisticated, computer-driven technologies based on superior imaging. They led to excellent visual outcome and very low toxicity that would jointly lead to completely abandoning the use of conventionally planned and executed (2D) RT from this setting.

7.1

Postoperative Radiation Therapy

Surgery and radiation therapy can be combined both ways, as either postoperative (adjuvant) radiotherapy or post-radiotherapy (adjuvant) surgery. While the majority of the data come from the postoperative setting, some of the recent reports indicated that surgery can be practiced in cases with severe, progressive visual loss and optic disk oedema not only before, but also after radiation therapy (Turbin et al. 2006).

Postoperative radiation therapy has traditionally followed surgery that had been described as either bi-

opsy or partial/subtotal resection or complete tumour resection. It has mostly been practiced in cases when primary ONSM extended to the intracranial sites with clearly documented visual impairment. In such cases, although there is presumably bigger bulk of the primary tumour, resection of both intraorbital and intracranial component of the disease should be attempted at the same time. Resection of as much tumour as possible should be an ideal goal. It should, however, be switched to a subtotal resection if no clear resection planes are identified around the optic nerve to minimize visual loss, if possible at all. In such cases postoperative RT was frequently administered.

Several studies at the end of the 1980s showed that this might be an effective approach (Ito et al. 1988; Kennerdell et al. 1988; Kupersmith et al. 1987). In a series of Kupersmith et al. (1987), there were three groups of patients treated between 1965 and 1984 at New York University Medical Center. One (group A; n = 4) had received radiation therapy as the primary

B. Jeremić, MD, PhD
International Atomic Energy Agency, Wagramer Strasse 5, P.O. Box 100, 1400 Vienna, Austria

mode of therapy; the second (group B; n = 4) consisted of patients undergoing radiation therapy for tumour recurrence with documented visual deterioration within 2 years of initial subtotal surgical resection; the third group (group C; n = 12) of patients underwent radiation therapy for residual tumour 1–2 months following subtotal surgical resection. All but one patient were treated with either a 4-MV linear accelerator or a cobalt 60 unit. Small fields were used, encompassing the tumour plus a limited margin. A dose of 50–55 Gy was given by means of two or three portals fractionated over 6 weeks. Only one patient was first evaluated following operation with >70 Gy given total dose. Majority of patients had primary tumours in the region of sphenoid wing, only one having orbital ONSM. Of four patients in the Group B, none had pONSM.

Ito et al. (1988) presented a series of 11 cases of intraorbital meningiomas with progressive visual disturbance for months and years. Seven cases were cases of primary orbital meningioma, while four cases were secondary orbital meningiomas. Of primary orbital meningiomas, three cases had no light perception at admission. Three cases had limitation of extraocular movement. No cases had enlargement of optic canal or other abnormalities on skull roentgenograms. In CT scans was seen a globular (n = 6) or a tubular (n = 1) mass in the retrobulbar perioptic region. Only three cases in this series underwent postoperative radiation therapy after either subtotal (n = 2) or partial (n = 1) resection of the tumour located either intraorbitally or intrecranially. Radiation therapy was given with 40–45 Gy. In two cases no change in visual fields and visual acuity was noted, while one patient improved in both visual fields and visual acuity.

Kennerdell et al. (1988) presented a series of 38 patients with 39 eyes which were either followed up by observation alone (n = 18), or treated with either radiation therapy (n = 6) or surgery only (n = 10) or treated with postoperative radiation therapy (n = 5). In the last group, three patients underwent subtotal excision. Radiation therapy was administered with the total dose of 55–60 Gy. In two of these patients, visual acuity and colour vision have been stable, with improved or stable visual fields for 6 and 9 years. The third patient underwent an orbital unroofing with partial excision of the meningioma. Because it was known at surgery that significant tumour remained, the patient underwent postoperative radiation therapy 2 months postoperatively, even though visual acuity was stable. Over an 8-year period, radiologic findings have remained stable, but visual acuity has decreased from 20/100 to 20/800. Two other patients underwent subtotal surgical excision of an ONSM not followed by

radiation therapy initially. In one patient, with a visual acuity of NLP because of an apical tumour, the orbital apex with optic nerve was removed via a craniotomy. Twenty years later, intracranial and sinus spread were noted but the patient refused further surgery and was treated with radiation therapy. After 3 years of follow-up, radiologic and clinical findings were stable. The second patient had subtotal removal of an ONSM and maintained with a visual acuity of 20/30 for 7 years, after which time visual acuity decreased to 20/50 with an increasing visual field defect. The patient then received 55 Gy of radiation and has maintained a visual acuity of 20/50 and a stable visual field for 6 years. In all 5 patients (follow up: range 3–9 years; median 6 years), no complications were observed with 2 patients improving their vision, while in 3 patients it remained unchanged.

In a series of Petty et al. (1985) a total of 12 patients with incompletely resected meningioma were postoperatively irradiated with tumour doses ranging from 4800 to 6080 cGy, using photons of 6, 18, or 25 MV. Only one patient had orbital meningioma. Radiation therapy dose in that patient was 5630 cGy used in 32 daily fractions in a total of 45 days. Progression-free period was 4.5 years with a good visual outcome reported. No toxicity was reported in that patient.

Turbin et al. (2002) presented 16 patients treated with postoperative radiotherapy, out of a total of 64 patients with ONSM. Only 2 patients underwent total resections, while 14 patients underwent biopsies or partial resections followed by postoperative radiation therapy. Radiation therapy dose ranged from 4000 to 5500 cGy using either conventional multiport or conformal external beam radiation therapy. Similarly to observation-only and surgery only groups of patients, patients treated with postoperative radiation therapy experienced statistically significant decrease in visual acuity. When comparing vision at diagnosis or at treatment to vision at last follow-up, 5 of 16 (31.3%) patients treated with surgery and postoperative radiation therapy showed at least two lines of improvement (including improvement from light perception to counting fingers etc.) that remained stable through the last follow-up, which was similar to radiation therapy alone patients, but in sharp contrast to surgery only patients. Complication rate was 62.5% in this group of patients. This included two cases of retinopathy/vascular occlusion, two cases of neovascular glaucoma, one case of cerebral infarct and concurrent cerebrospinal fluid leak, two cases of severe motility deficit, one case of persistent iritis, one case of recurrent orbital haemorrhage, and one case of lymphoma). Authors speculated that it was difficult to assess if a combination therapy increased the susceptibility to treatment complications because of varied therapies and surgical approaches.

In the study of Saeed et al. (2003), with a total of 88 patients, there were 6 patients undergoing primary radiotherapy. Five had between 50 and 55 Gy in 28–30 daily fractions, and 1 underwent stereotactic fractionated conformal radiation therapy with a linear accelerator in 28 daily fractions for a total of 45 Gy. In an addition to these, 11 patients which underwent orbitotomy for biopsy alone, 4 of which underwent postoperative radiation therapy. In addition, three patients underwent tumour debulking followed by radiation therapy. Although the follow up for these three patients was rather limited (less than 2 years), no signs of recurrence had been detected. Contrary to specifications of radiation therapy characteristics in patients treated with primary radiation therapy, unfortunately, no specification of radiation therapy characteristics was offered in patients treated with postoperative radiation therapy.

These series have sometimes covered prolonged periods of time during which surgical procedures varied. However, radiation therapy characteristics have also changed even more. In particular, initial studies were simply planned, mostly two-dimensionally (2D). More recent publications also included CT-based treatment planning and only a few patients have been treated with either 3D CRT or SFRT (Turbin et al. 2006). These discrepancies, in addition to very small patient numbers, and frequently lacking clear time-dose-fractionation pattern of radiation therapy regimens used, make any conclusion regarding the radiation therapy impact rather impossible.

However, summarizing the data, Dutton (1992) noted that in these, rather small, series improved vision ranged from 33% to 44%, stable vision ranged from 25% to 67%, while decreased vision ranged from 0% to 31%. More recent studies (Turbin et al. 2002) confirmed this observation. This approach, however, is associated with high rate of postoperative complications. Combination of less aggressive surgery and postoperative RT did not lead to substantially lower incidence of postoperative complications when compared to surgery alone (Turbin et al. 2002). Coupled with the most recent data on the effectiveness of modern RT alone (Pitz et al. 2002; Liu et al. 2002; Becker et al. 2002a; Baumert et al. 2004; Richards et al. 2005; Landert et al. 2005; Sitathanee et al. 2006; Paridaens et al. 2006; Andrews et al. 2002; Moyer et al. 2000; Narayan et al. 2003; Eng et al. 1992; Lee et al. 1996; Klink et al. 1998; Grant and Cain 1998, Fineman and Augsburger 1999; Uy et al. 2002), especially those of stereotactic fractionated radiation therapy (Pitz et al. 2002; Liu et al. 2002; Becker et al. 2002a; Baumert et al.

2004; Richards et al. 2005; Landert et al. 2005; Sitathanee et al. 2006; Paridaens et al. 2006; Andrews et al. 2002), these data warrant re-evaluation of this approach in order to identify a subgroup of patients, which may benefit from this approach. Contrary to primary ONSM, secondary ONSM seem as the most likely candidate for combined surgery and postoperative RT, regardless of the extent of surgery and the type of RT employed.

However, a recent publication of Turbin et al. (2006) re-examined the role of surgery as an adjuvant therapy in patients with ONSM. Two patients which presented with unilateral ONSM were discussed. In the first patient, progressive visual loss and disc oedema had been observed after previously administered SFRT, while the second patient was subsequently treated with SFRT after decompression surgery. SFRT was used with 5040 cGy given over 28 daily sessions in 37 days in the first patient. Total radiation therapy dose of 5040 cGy was given over 6 weeks using five-field 3D conformal radiation therapy (3D CRT) in the second patient. After excision of a dural window and biopsy of the tumour from the nerve sheath, visual acuity improved, both coinciding with resolution of disc oedema Visual acuity and visual fields in both patients remained stable after initial improvement for the period of 3.5 and 7 years, respectively. No orbital tumour spread had occurred in both patients. The cause of the post-irradiation visual loss in the first patient was judged to be nerve compression within a tight sheath, which led the optic nerve head congestion and macular oedema. Furthermore, the lack of further progression after surgical intervention supported that the course was not consistent with radiation-induced neuropathy or retinopathy. In the second case, a nerve sheath decompression and biopsy in the form of removal of extruding tumour was performed because of the rapidly worsening clinical course and continued radiographic debate concerning the differential diagnosis of the lesion. The surgery, which decompressed the orbital nerve within its sheath ultimately contributed to restoration of vision despite a prolonged episode of non-light perception confirmed by two preoperative and one postoperative examination. The postoperative return of vision justified the subsequent treatment with fractionated conformal stereotactic radiation therapy. Although both patients underwent steroid treatment as well, the surgical intervention was the likely cause of that improvement, rather than other components of therapy. The authors concluded that although SFRT is being increasingly used alone in pONSM with great success, there may be a selected subset of patients with prominent disc oedema and associated severe and rapidly progressive visual loss that could benefit from partial optic nerve decompression by fenestration as adjuvant vision-preserving therapy.

In an era of important advances in imaging and radiation therapy, the role of combined surgery and radiation therapy, given either post- or pre-operatively or for recurrences, remain of minor importance. Only in selected cases can it be considered as valuable treatment option. It will continue depending on developments of both imaging and radiation therapy. In particular, with prolonged follow-up periods, investigators would be able to determinate more precisely the place and the role of combined treatment modality in this setting.

7.2
Exclusive Conventional Radiation Therapy

The first mentioning of radiation therapy alone in ONSM can be found in the report of Byers (1914), who credited McReynolds with the first use of this treatment modality. It also seems that it was actually Smith et al. (1981) who were first to document clearly the effectiveness of RT in pONSM some 70 years later! In the report of Smith et al. (1981), single-institution experience (1975–1981) on the use of radiation therapy in selected cases of ONSM was reviewed. Documentation of the results in five patients seems to have been the very first systematic approach to address the place and the role of external beam radiation therapy in this setting. All five patients had various degrees of visual acuity and visual field impairment in the preceding periods (before radiation therapy had been instituted). There was no standard policy of radiation therapy administered. The total doses administered were 5300 cGy, 200 cGy plus 5220 cGy, 3600 cGy, 4140 cGy and 5400 cGy, respectively with a variety of treatment field arrangements such as two parallel, coplanar opposing fields, or a combination of a straight perpendicular field and a lateral field. Gross tumour volume directed field sizes and inclusion of different portions of the orbit or optic canal. Fractionation was mostly standard (175–200 cGy per fraction). Although not specified, it is safe to assume than none of these patients underwent CT-based treatment planning. Regardless of these facts that one can see as shortcoming nowadays, functional outcome was rather impressive. Visual acuity and visual fields improved in all four non-blind patients, while in the one blind patient, they eye was reportedly less tender to touch, and there had been no signs of progression of proptosis on that eye. It led authors to conclude that "although radiation therapy may only help palliate the patient's vision for perhaps 2 years or so, this form of treatment

definitely warrants further consideration". Although no radiation therapy-related toxicity was reported in their study, authors suggested even smaller total dose – in the region of 4000 cGy – due to presumed responsiveness of pONSMs to radiation therapy. Authors went even further on to claim that in cases with progressive vision loss with acuity down to the 20/80–20/200 level, optic atrophy, optocilliary veins, and with appropriate neuro-radiologic and CT findings, a course of radiation therapy can be given without biopsy or surgical intervention in *selected* cases. It remained, however, unknown, how *selected* cases would be distinguished from other cases of pONSM and based on which criteria, some of which may have been specified above.

In the study of Sarkies (1987), of a total of 22 patients with ONSMs, two patients with bilateral ONSM were treated with radiation therapy to orbits when visual acuity began to decline in their only seeing eye. One patient had 1325 cGy to both orbits in four fractions, but radiation therapy was terminated because his vision declined during the radiation therapy course. The other patient received 4000 cGy to both orbits and chiasm in 12 treatments. There was no improvement in acuity, but 2 months after radiation therapy ended the visual field had improved slightly. Unfortunately, the visual field declined further within the next 2 months. In the light of his experience in two patients, Sarkies (1987) questioned the use of radiation therapy in this setting likely because his results simply did not repeat that of Smith et al. (1981). Again, no radiation therapy specifics, other than fractionation data, were provided and it remained unknown whether there were any treatment-related toxicities.

Although none of the four patients with meningioma of the anterior visual pathway in the study of Kupersmith et al. (1987) had pONSM, after external beam radiation therapy with doses of 5000–5500 cGy delivered using small fields from a 4-MV linear accelerator, visual acuity post radiation therapy improved in all four patients. Visual fields were improved in three patients while the fourth patient remained unchanged.

In the study of Kennerdell et al. (1988), radiation therapy was used in six patients with ONSM confined to the orbit. There were 4 females and 2 males with their age ranging from 49 to 81 years (median 59.5 years). All patients had progressive visual field loss or decreasing visual acuity before radiation therapy. Visual acuity counting fingers at 2 feet ranged around 20/40 with the median being 20/60. Colour vision tested using Ishihara colour plates ranged from 0/8 to 4/8 with the median of 0/8. Visual fields description pre-radiotherapy included cecocentral scotoma in four patients, superior and inferior arcuate defects in one patient and nasal island in one patient. Radiation therapy was administered with tumour doses of 5400–5500 cGy given in 28–32 daily fractions. After follow-up that ranged from 3 to 7 years (median 6 years), all patients improved visual acuity and visual fields, while two out of six patients improved their colour vision. The improved visual function has been maintained for 30–84 months. No patient has shown decreased visual function or tumour growth on computed tomography. In no case tumour shrinkage had been observed on either CT and/or MRI after radiation therapy. The only complication observed was a transient dry eye in one patient. Unfortunately, no additional radiation therapy specifications were provided such as dose prescription, choice of radiation portals, etc.

In the study of ITO et al. (1988), 2 out of a total of 11 patients with ONSM were treated with radiation therapy alone. Symptoms lasted for 2 and 7 years in the two globular-appearing ONSM before radiation therapy had been administered for progressive vision loss. Radiation therapy doses were 40 and 60 Gy, respectively. After 2–2.5 years of follow-up, both patients' visual fields and visual acuity improved with no treatment related toxicity being documented in these two cases.

In other sporadic reports, RT doses of mostly around 5500 cGy were used reporting favourable outcomes (ROOTMAN 1988). When DUTTON (1992) summarized some of the data available from the literature (in a total of 12 presented pONSM patients), visual acuity improved in 75%, remained stable in 8%, and declined in 17%, after the follow-up periods of 2–6 years. The effectiveness of RT alone in ONSM were documented in only a few patients, coupled with both the belief that meningiomas are radioresistant (DYKE and DAVIDOFF 1942; SIMPSON 1957) and the fear of excessive toxicity were the major factors preventing wider application of RT in pONSM. Indeed, in these early reports, RT-induced toxicity in patients with ONSM was documented. RT techniques used at that time included either lateral or wedged-pair RT fields based on two-dimensional CT-based treatment planning, when it became available. Before that, it was based on pure anatomical radiography-based planning, and not based on sophisticated computer-driven algorithms of RT dose planning and delivery. Not surprisingly, this has been considered now for more than 20 years as an inferior planning and treatment approach that may have inevitably led to complications of anterior visual pathway and brain parenchyma. With the time, however, RT-induced toxicity was largely demystified. It was observed that brain necrosis is extremely unusual after 54 Gy given in 1.8-Gy daily fractions, being 0.2% in an analysis, which included 1388 patients (BECKER et al. 2002b). It was also observed that the risk of injury to the optic pathways depends on the single and total RT doses. Without previous surgical damage to the pathways, with the single dose of < 2.0 Gy and the total dose ranging from 45 to 50 Gy, this risk was about < 2% (BECKER et al. 2002b; BRADA et al. 1993). If the total dose increases to 54 Gy, the risk of neuropathy after RT of meningioma is < 5% (GOLDSMITH et al. 1992; PARSONS et al. 1994). However, in the study on head and neck cancer (PARSONS et al. 1994), with the dose of < 59 Gy no injury was observed in 106 optic nerves. With >60 Gy, the 15-year actuarial risk of developing optic neuropathy was 47% with fraction sizes of >1.9 Gy, but was only 11% with fraction sizes < 1.9 Gy, indicating an important influence of the dose per fraction.

The more recent series occasionally included a mixture of patients: some treated with conventionally planned and executed (2D) radiation therapy, some with 3D radiation therapy. In the study of TURBIN et al. (2002), a total of 34 out of 64 patients with ONSM were treated with radiation therapy alone. For the 33 patients with known dosimetric data, total tumour doses ranged from 4000 to 4500 cGy (5 patients), or from 5000 to 5100 cGy (14 patients) and from 5400 to 5500 cGy (14 patients). In most of these patients, either conventionally planned multiport radiation therapy was instituted, or some patients (in the more recent years preceding the publication) were treated using 3D conformal radiation therapy. No details were given on possible differences in the outcome and toxicity pattern between the two groups of patients treated exclusively with RT (2D vs 3D). Visual outcome included 44.4% of patients showing at least two lines of improvement; six (33%) patients experienced toxicity which included four patients experiencing retinopathy, one patients experiencing persistent iritis and one patient experiencing temporal lobe atrophy. It again remained unknown whether perhaps more sophisticated treatment planning and delivery (3D) may have led to lower incidence of toxicity than did 2D radiation therapy.

More recently, SAEED et al. (2003) provided the data on 6 patients undergoing radiation therapy (out of a total of 88 patients treated at the University of British Columbia and the University of Amsterdam). Five patients underwent radiation therapy with total tumour doses between 50 and 55 Gy in 28–30 daily fractions. Four of the five patients had a follow-up of between 3 and 5 years, and two less than 1 year. Before radiation therapy, all patients demonstrated progressive deterioration of visual acuity and visual fields. All have improved after radiation therapy and none have shown either a decrease in visual function or tumour growth on imaging. The only complication seen was post-irradiation cataract and subsequent macular degeneration in one patient.

In summary, although conventional radiation therapy provided good results in patients with pONSM, these data must be considered along the more recent, 3D conformal and stereotactic radiation therapy achievements in this disease. Having obtained good results, the latter two techniques have major advantage over more traditional 2D radiation therapy. This is so regarding both tumour control and toxicity. Both issues are superiorly addressed by more sophisticated, computer-driven technologies based on superior imaging. They led to excellent visual outcome and very low toxicity that would jointly lead to completely abandoning the use of conventionally planned and executed (2D) radiation therapy from this setting.

References

Andrews DW, Faroozan R, Yang BP et al. (2002) Fractionated stereotactic radiotherapy for the treatment of optic nerve sheath meningiomas: preliminary observations of 33 optic nerves in 30 patients with historical comparison to observation with or without prior surgery. Neurosurgery 51:890–904

Baumert BG, Villa S, Studer G, Mirimanoff R-O et al. (2004) Early improvements in vision after fractionated stereotactic radiotherapy for primary optic nerve sheath meningioma. Radiother Oncol 72:169–174

Becker G, Jeremic B, Pitz S et al. (2002a) Stereotactic fractionated radiotherapy in patients with optic nerve sheath meningioma. Int J Radiat Oncol Biol Phys 54:1422–1429

Becker G, Kocher M, Kortmann RD et al. (2002b) Radiation therapy in the multimodal treatment approach of pituitary adenoma. Strahlenther Onkol 178:173–186

Brada M, Rajan B, Traish D et al. (1993) The long-term efficacy of conservative surgery and radiotherapy in the control of pituitary adenomas. Clin Endocrinol 38:571–578

Byers WGM (1914) Tumors of the optic nerve. JAMA 63:20–25

Dutton JJ (1992) Optic nerve sheath meningioma. Surv Ophthalmol 37:167–183

Dyke CG, Davidoff LM (1942) Roentgen treatment of diseases of the nervous system. Lea and Febiger, Philadelphia, p 113

Eng T, Albright N, Kuwahara G et al. (1992) Precision radiation therapy for optic nerve sheath meningiomas. Int J Radiat Oncol Biol Phys 22:1093–1098

Fineman MS, Augsburger JJ (1999) A new approach to an old problem. Surv Ophthalmol 3:519–524

Goldsmith BJ, Rosenthal SA, Wara WM, Larson DA (1992) Optic neuropathy after irradiation of meningioma. Radiology 185:71–76

Grant W III, Cain RB (1998) Intensity modulated conformal therapy for intracranial lesions. Med Dosim 2 3:237–241

Ito M, Ishizawa A, Miyaoka M, Sato K, Ishii S (1988) Intraorbital meningiomas. Surgical management and role of radiation therapy. Surg Neurol 29:448–453

Kennerdell JS, Maroon JC, Malton M, Warren FA (1988) The management of optic nerve sheath meningiomas. Am J Ophthalmol 106:450–457

Klink DF, Miller NR, Williams J (1998) Preservation of residual vision 2 years after stereotactic radiosurgery for a presumed optic nerve sheath meningioma. J Neuro-Ophthalmol 18:117–120

Kupersmith MJ, Warren FA, Newall J, Ransohoff J (1987) Irradiation of meningiomas of the intracranial anterior visual pathway. Ann Neurol 21:131–137

Landert M, Baumert B, Bosch MM, Lutolf U, Landau K (2005) The visual impact of fractionated stereotactic conformal radiotherapy on seven eyes with optic nerve sheath meningiomas. J Neuro-Ophthalmol 25:86–91

Lee AG, Woo SY, Miller NR, Safran AB, Grant WH, Butler EB (1996) Improvement in visual function in an eye with a presumed optic nerve sheath meningioma after treatment with three-dimensional conformal irradiation therapy. J Neuro-Ophthalmol 16:247–251

Liu JK, Forman S, Hershewe GL, Moorthy CR, Benzil DL (2002) Optic nerve sheath meningiomas: visual improvement after stereotactic radiotherapy. Neurosurgery 50:950–957

Moyer PD, Golnik KC, Breneman J (2000) Treatment of optic nerve sheath meningioma with three-dimensional conformal radiation. Am J Ophthalmol 129:694–696

Narayan S, Cornblath WT, Sandler HM et al. (2003) Preliminary visual outcomes after three-dimensional conformal ration therapy fort optic nerve sheath meningioma. Int J Radiat Oncol Biol Phys 56:537–543

Paridaens ADA, van Ruyven RLJ, Eijkenboom WMH, Mooy CM, van den Bosch WA (2006) Stereotactic irradiation of biopsy proved optic nerve sheath meningioma. Br J Ophthalmol 246–247

Parsons JT, Bova FJ, Fitzgerald CR, Mendenhall WM, Million RR (1994) Radiation optic neuropathy after megavoltage external-beam irradiation: analysis of time-dose factors. Int J Radiat Oncol Biol Phys 30:755–763

Petty AM, Kun LE, Meyer GA (1985) Radiation therapy for incompletely resected meningiomas. J Neurosurg 62:502–507

Pitz S, Becker G, Schiefer U et al. (2002) Stereotactic fractionated irradiation of optic nerve sheath meningioma: a new treatment alternative. Br J Ophthalmol 86:1265–1268

Richards JC, Roden D, Harper CS (2005) Management of sight-threatening optic nerve sheath meningioma with fractionated stereotactic radiotherapy. Clin Experimen Ophthalmol 33:137–141

Rootman J (1988) Diseases of the orbit. A multidisciplinary approach, JB Lippincott, London, pp 281–285

Saeed P, Rootman J, Nugent RA, White VA, Mackenzie IR, Koornnef L (2003) Optic nerve sheath meningiomas. Ophthalmology 110:2019–2030

Sarkies NJC (1987) Optic nerve sheath meningioma: diagnostic features and therapeutic alternatives. Eye 1:597–602

Simpson D (1957) Recurrence of intracranial meningiomas after surgical treatment. J Neurol Neurosurg Psychaitr 20:22–39

Sitathanee C, Dhanachai M, Poonyathalang A, Tuntiyatorn L, Theerapancharoen S (2006) Stereotactic radiation therapy for optic nerve sheath meningioma: an experience at Ramathibodi hospital. J Med Assoc Thai 89:1665–1669

Smith JL, Vuksanovic MM, Yates BM, Bienfang DC (1981) Radiation therapy for primary optic nerve meningiomas. J Clin Neuro-ophthalmol 1:85–99

Turbin RE, Thompson CR, Kennerdell JS, Cockerham KP, Kupersmith MJ (2002) A long-term visual outcome comparison in patients with optic nerve sheath meningioma managed with observation, surgery, radiotherapy, or surgery and radiotherapy. Ophthalmology 109:890–899

Turbin RE, Wladis EJ, Frohman LP, Langer PD, Kennerdell JS (2006) Role of surgery as adjuvant therapy in optic nerve sheath meningioma. Ophthalm Plast Reconstruct Surg 22(4):278–282

Uy NW, Woo SY, The BS et al. (2002) Intensity-modulated radiation therapy (IMRT) for meningioma. Int J Radiat Oncol Biol Phys 53:1265–1270

3D Conformal RT

Simon S. Lo, Samuel T. Chao, and John H. Suh

8

CONTENTS

KEY POINTS

Optic nerve sheath meningiomas (ONSM) are rare tumors that account for 1%–2% of all meningiomas. Radiation therapy (RT) is regarded as the treatment of choice for patients with ONSM when serviceable vision is still present. Data in the literature show promising results with the use of RT for ONSM. Apart from tumor control, improvement of vision can also be observed. Before the advent of three-dimensional (3D) image-based planning, critical structures such as the optic nerves, optic chiasm, pituitary, and eyes as well as normal brain parenchyma frequently received a high dose of radiation leading to a greater risk for acute and late complications. With the use of 3D conformal RT, the tumor and those critical structures can be accurately outlined. Improved tumor coverage and sparing of critical structures can be readily achieved. The published data on the use of 3D conformal RT for ONSM documenting its efficacy and limited toxicity is sparse. Meticulous treatment planning is necessary to optimize the therapeutic ratio.

S. S. Lo, MD
Associate Professor of Radiation Medicine and Neurosurgery, Director of Residency in Radiation Oncology, Director of Neuro-Radiation Oncology and Stereotactic Radiation Therapy, Department of Radiation Medicine, Arthur G. James Cancer Hospital, Ohio State University Medical Center, 300 West 1st Avenue, Ste 088a , Columbus, OH 43210, USA

S. T. Chao, MD
Cleveland Clinic, Brain Tumor and Neuro-Oncology Center, Department of Radiation Oncology, T 28, Cleveland, OH 44195, USA

J. H. Suh, MD
Cleveland Clinic, Brain Tumor and Neuro-Oncology Center, Department of Radiation Oncology, T 28, Cleveland, OH 44195, USA

8.1
Introduction

Optic nerve sheath meningiomas (ONSM) are rare tumors and account for 1%–2% of all meningiomas (Baumert et al. 2004). Most optic nerve meningiomas (ONSM) are not surgically resectable without causing a substantial risk of visual deterioration because dissection of the pial vascular supply of the nerve is often unavoidable (Dutton 1992). Radiation therapy is regarded as the treatment of choice in most cases of

ONSM where patients still have serviceable vision. Data in the literature on the use of primary radiotherapy (RT) show promising results (MELIAN and JAY 2004). Despite the notion that meningiomas tend to give slow response and minimal shrinkage, RT can prevent or delay tumor progression and visual improvement has been observed after treatment. Secondary to the concerns of radiation-induced complications, expectant observation has been advocated. Radiation-induced complications are determined by the dose delivered and the volume of the normal brain parenchyma or critical structures irradiated. In the two-dimensional (2D) era where treatment planning was performed using plain radiographs, a substantial amount of brain parenchyma and critical structures would be treated to the prescribed dose. With the advent of three-dimensional (3D) treatment planning, it is possible to generate a conformal radiation dose distribution around the target volume while sparing normal brain parenchyma and critical structures. This chapter will discuss various aspects of 3D conformal RT for the treatment of ONSM.

8.2
Principles and Techniques of 3D Conformal RT

Three-dimensional conformal RT entails irradiation of the patient from multiple beam directions. As opposed to 2D RT, the beams utilized in 3D CRT are conformally shaped to the tumor or the planning treatment volume (PTV) and are non-opposing and sometimes non-co-planar. This process is facilitated by virtual simulation utilizing a treatment planning computerized tomography (CT). The isocenter is usually placed in the center of the PTV. For each individual beam, the intervening superficial normal tissue will receive a higher dose than the isocenter. However, when the composite of all the beams of a 3D conformal RT plan is generated, the PTV will receive a much higher dose than the surrounding or superficial tissue. The most important components of 3D conformal RT include immobilization, target delineation, and treatment planning. These aspects will be discussed below.

8.2.1
Immobilization

To achieve excellent precision of radiation treatment delivery, the use of a proper immobilization device is of utmost importance. Because ONSM are surrounded by critical structures such as the optic chiasm, ipsilateral

eye including cornea and lens, ipsilateral lacrimal gland, and pituitary, a modest deviation of treatment position can result in significant increase of the radiation dose delivered to those structures. Furthermore, because of the highly conformal dose distribution around the PTV, a shift larger than the amount accounted for by the PTV expansion will result in a marginal miss which may jeopardize tumor control. Colleagues from University of California, San Francisco (UCSF) have demonstrated that with proper use of a mask for immobilization, only 2.5% of the setups were more than 0.5 cm compared to 21% when a mask was not used for setup (ENG et al. 1992).

Depending on the technique used, the position of the patient's head can be manipulated to facilitate RT treatment planning and delivery. Colleagues from UCSF described a 3D conformal RT technique where the patient's head was rotated contralaterally by 15–27° and the neck flexion adjusted to align the affected optic nerve to a line perpendicular to the horizontal plane (ENG et al. 1992). The patient's head was immobilized using a head support, a thermoplastic mask that was formed to the head, and a frame that locked the mask and head in a reproducible position. This setup arrangement facilitated the technique utilizing two superior lateral and vertex beams. The details of this technique are discussed later in this chapter. Alternatively, the patient's head can be placed in a neutral position in a thermoplastic mask or locked with a thermoplastic mask onto a reclining head board (Fig. 8.1). The main advantage of immobilization of the patient's head on a reclining head board is that the vertex beam will not exit through the thyroid in the neck and the trunk.

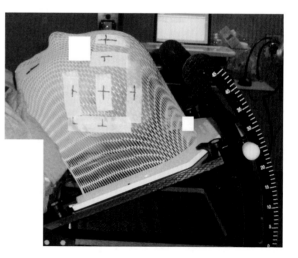

Fig. 8.1. The patient's head is locked with a thermoplastic mask onto a reclining head board

The use of a relocatable stereotactic headframe can improve the setup accuracy and will be discussed in another chapter of this book.

8.2.2
Target Delineation

Meningiomas are extra-axial tumors that do not have blood-brain barrier. They typically enhance on T1 with gadolinium sequence of magnetic resonance imaging (MRI). The extent of an ONSM can be obscured by the marrow fat of the skull bone and the orbital fat. Therefore, a fat suppression sequence is most helpful demonstrating the lesion. The MRI is usually fused with a treatment planning contrast CT to facilitate target delineation. The gross tumor volume (GTV) is defined by the intense contrast enhancement on CT or MRI. Overall, MRI is superior to CT for determination of GTV, but CT can be used in patients not suitable for MRI. If MRI-defined GTV is not completely inclusive of the treatment planning CT-defined GTV, the composite GTV may be used.

In the 2D era, a 2-cm margin was typically placed the tumor or GTV to avoid a geographic miss. With the availability of modern imaging, it is possible to precisely delineate the GTV. Most ONSM are World Health Or-

ganisation (WHO) class 1 meningiomas which typically have sharp margins of demarcation from the surrounding tissue. Therefore, a margin expansion is not necessary to generate a clinical target volume (CTV). Hence, the CTV is equivalent to the GTV. To account for daily set-up variation, an extra margin is created around the GTV to generate a planning treatment volume (PTV). When a thermoplastic mask is used, a margin expansion of 0.3–0.5 cm is used to generate a PTV (Fig. 8.2). If a relocatable stereotactic headframe such as a Gill-Thomas-Cosman headframe is used, the margin expansion can be decreased to 0.2 cm. Stereotactic radiation therapy for ONSM is discussed in a later chapter of this book. Apart from the delineation of GTV and PTV, several critical structures such as the eyes, lens, optic chiasm. optic nerves, pituitary, lacrimal glands, brainstem, spinal cord, and thyroid are contoured, so that efforts can be made to block those structures. Furthermore, dose volume histograms of those structures can be generated, so that the therapeutic ratio of each plan can be assessed.

8.2.3
Treatment Planning

With proper immobilization and accurate target delineation, high quality 3D conformal RT can be facilitated by careful treatment planning. The goals of 3D conformal RT for the treatment of ONSM are to adequately cover the PTV while minimizing the radiation dose to the normal brain parenchyma and other critical structures. Efforts should be made to avoid any beams passing or exiting through the eyes, the lacrimal glands, and the pituitary gland. Since the involved optic nerve is encased by the ONSM which is included within the PTV, any hotspots inside the PTV should be minimized or avoided. This can be achieved by using beam modifiers such as wedges, different beam weighting, and sometimes higher beam energy.

The design of the treatment portal shapes and selection of treatment beam directions are performed using a specialized computer display called beam's eye view (BEV) which shows all the contoured structures such as brainstem, spinal cord, eyes, optic nerve, optic chiasm, lenses, lacrimal glands, and pituitary from any desired beam direction. The utilization of BEV is beneficial in limiting the radiation doses to various critical structures to below the acceptable constraints. The optimization of the radiation beams or forward planning is performed through manual manipulation. Wedges can be added to modulate the beam intensity in one dimension. After the beam shapes, beam directions, beam weighting, and

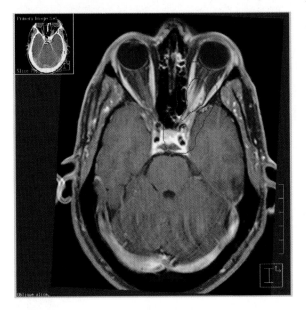

Fig. 8.2. On the T1 sequence of the MRI, the contrast-enhanced primary ONSM is encasing the left optic nerve; both the ONSM and the portion of the optic nerve encased by the tumor are included as the GTV (*inner contour*); the PTV (*outer contour*) is created by a margin expansion to account for daily set-up variations

wedging are finalized, a computer plan is then generated. The resultant isodose distribution can be visualized in axial, coronal, and sagittal planes. Resultant
dose-volume histograms (DVHs) of all the contoured
structures are generated to evaluate the dose-volume
relationships of and the maximum dose delivered to
those structures. If either the isodose distribution or
DVHs are not satisfactory, the beam parameters can be
adjusted before recalculating the resultant isodose distribution. It is important to examine the isodose distribution in axial, coronal, and sagittal planes as well as the
DVHs of the critical structures when a 3D conformal
RT plan is evaluated.

The proper selection of treatment beams is crucial
in the generation of an excellent 3D conformal RT plan.
Orientation of the treatment beams is chosen such that
the PTV is well separated from the organs-at-risk.

In terms of the radiation dose, the typical prescription is 50.4–54 Gy in 1.8-Gy fractions. Data in the literature on meningioma suggest that good local control can
be achieved with these dose regimens (LEE et al. 1996;
MOYER et al. 2000; BECKER et al. 2002; TURBIN et al.

2002; NARAYAN et al. 2003; BAUMERT et al. 2004; ME-
LIAN and JAY 2004; LANDERT et al. 2005; VAGEFI et al.
2006; LITRE et al. 2007). Based on the data from UCSF,
the optic apparatus can tolerate 54 Gy in 1.8-Gy fractions with low incidence of optic neuropathy (GOLD-
SMITH et al. 1992).

8.2.4
Treatment Techniques

As mentioned above, non-opposing and non-coplanar
beams are often used to achieve a better conformality.
Pertaining to ONSM, the location of the PTV in the orbital region limits the use of treatment beams aiming
from posteriorly because posterior or posterior oblique
beams can potentially exit through the ipsilateral or
contralateral eye. Therefore, beam directions are limited
to from the top and from the anterior and lateral directions. This section pertains to the different treatment
techniques used in 3D conformal RT for the treatment
of ONSM.

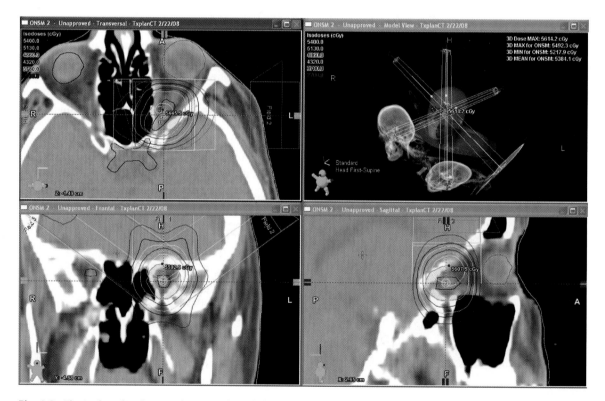

Fig. 8.3. The isodose distribution of a 3D conformal RT plan
similar to the technique described by colleagues from UCSF is
shown in axial, coronal, and sagittal planes; all the beams are
coming from the superior aspect of the head; effective sparing
of the ipsilateral eye, optic chiasm and pituitary is achieved;
however, more normal brain parenchyma is included in the
high dose zone

The earliest 3D conformal RT technique was described by the colleagues from UCSF and this has been described earlier (ENG et al. 1992). The technique utilizes three beams all from the superior direction (vertex and right and left superior obliques) and allows effective sparing of the ipsilateral eye, optic chiasm and pituitary. The contralateral eye and optic nerve can also be spared. However, because all the beams are coming from above, more normal brain parenchyma will be included in the high dose zone. Figure 8.3 demonstrates a 3D conformal RT technique similar to that described by the colleagues from UCSF except that a lateral head rotation was not used.

Alternatively, a three-beam arrangement can be used utilizing a vertex beam and two inferior oblique beams. Compared to the technique described in the previous paragraph, this technique yields a better conformality of the 95% isodose line to the PTV. However, one of the inferior oblique beams is coming from the contralateral side; therefore, the contralateral optic nerve and the pituitary are receiving a higher percentage of the dose prescribed to the PTV. Furthermore, the intermediate percentage isodose line include a larger amount of normal brain parenchyma. Figure 8.4 demonstrates the isodose distribution of this technique.

To achieve the best conformality around the PTV without "spilling" intermediate doses of radiation to the critical structures and normal brain parenchyma, a 3D conformal RT technique utilizing a larger number of non-coplanar and non-opposing beams can be used. With the use of larger number of beams coming from different non-coplanar directions, it is important to verify that there is no collision of the gantry with the patient or the treatment couch. Figure 8.5 demonstrates the isodose distribution for a 3D conformal RT plan utilizing six non-opposing and non-coplanar beams.

If micro-MLC is not available for beam shaping, a better conformality can be achieved using customized cerrobend blocks. Compared to MLC with 1-cm leaves, cerrobend blocks can achieve better beam shaping and hence better conformality around the PTV. Figure 8.6 demonstrates the difference between the use of MLC with 1-cm leaves and cerrobend blocks for beam shaping.

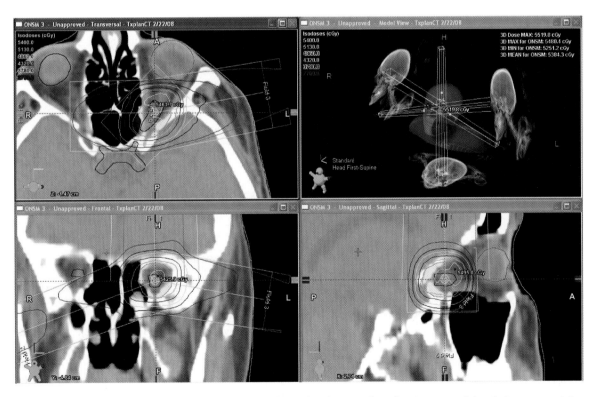

Fig. 8.4. The isodose distribution of a 3D conformal RT plan utilizing a different beam arrangement is shown in axial, coronal, and sagittal planes; a vertex and two inferior oblique beams are used; the conformality of the 95% line is improved but the contralateral optic nerve and the pituitary are receiving a higher percentage of the dose prescribed to the PTV and the intermediate percentage isodose line include a larger amount of normal brain parenchyma

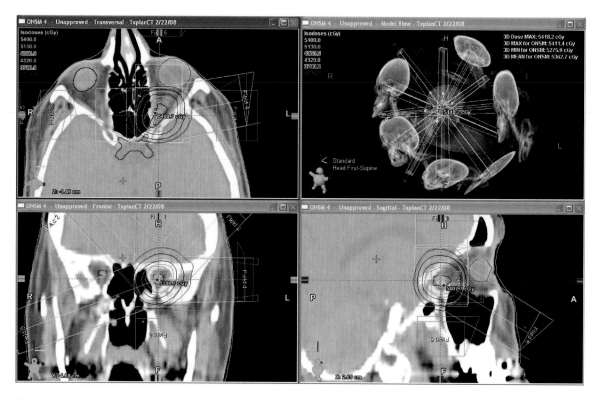

Fig. 8.5. The isodose distribution of a 3D conformal RT plan utilizing a larger number of non-coplanar and non-opposing beams is shown in axial, coronal, and sagittal planes; a high conformality of the 95% line around the PTV is achieved and the "spilling" of intermediate doses to critical structures and normal brain parenchyma can be minimized

8.3
Literature on 3D Conformal RT for ONSM

Although there is fair amount of literature on the use of radiation therapy for ONSM, most of the studies pertain to 2D radiation therapy or fractionated stereotactic radiotherapy.

Moyer et al. reported the treatment outcome of a patient with ONSM treated with 3D conformal RT (MOYER et al. 2000). The patient was a 35-year-old female with a 1.8 × 1.8 × 1.2-cm left ONSM that encased the left optic nerve. A radiation dose of 50.4 Gy in 28 fractions was given using 3D conformal RT. One month after treatment, the best corrected visual acuity improved form 20/200 to 20/40 and the visual field defect nearly com-

pletely disappeared. The optic nerve head edema also resolved. Subsequent follow-up at 4, 8, and 24 months showed further improvement of best corrected visual acuity to 20/30. Repeat MRI showed slight shrinkage of the ONSM. In another case report from Baylor College of Medicine, the patient with ONSM treated with 3D conformal RT had a similar outcome (LEE et al. 1996). In a study by TURBIN et al. (2002) the treatment outcomes of patients with ONSM were compared according to treatment. Out of the 34 patients were treated with RT with or without surgery (some with 2D and some with 3D conformal RT) to doses ranging from 40 to 55 Gy, only 2 patients showed radiographic progression. The tumor control rate with RT was much better compared to surgery alone. For the 18 patients who had RT only, eight (44.4%) patients showed at least 2 lines of

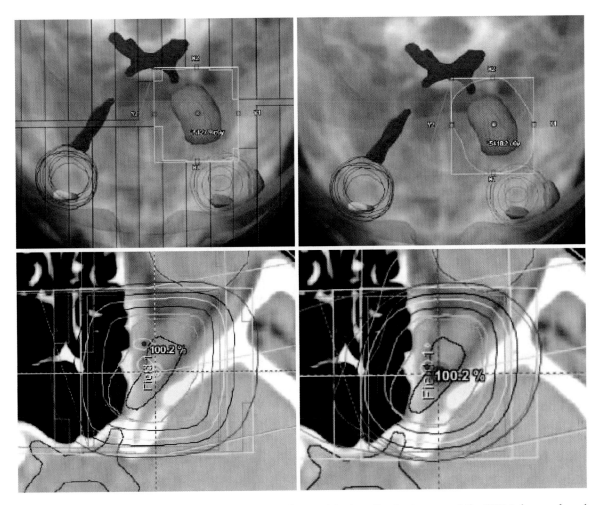

Fig. 8.6. In the *upper row*, beam shaping using MLC with 1-cm leaves (*left*) and cerrobend block (*right*) is compared; in the *lower row*, the resultant isodose distribution of the same plan using MLC (*left*) and cerrobend blocks is compared; the 95% isodose distribution around the PTV is less conformal with the use of MLC with 1-cm leaves compared to cerrobend blocks

improvement compared to 31.3% for patients who had surgery and RT.

NARAYAN et al. (2003) from University of Michigan reported their treatment results of 14 patients (1 male and 13 female) with ONSM treated with 3D conformal RT. The mean age of those patients was 44 years (range, 14–65 years). All patients presented with visual symptoms including decreased visual acuity (n = 13), visual field cut (n = 2), and proptosis (n = 2). Average duration of symptoms was 36 months. Median follow-up was 51.3 months (range, 8.9–80.9 months). Only one patient had surgery prior to 3D conformal RT. Of the 14 patients, 9 had visual acuity of 20/50 or better and 2 had visual acuity of 20/100. Target delineation was done using diagnostic MRI fused to treatment planning CT. The GTV was defined as the contrast enhanced tu-mor. A 1-cm expansion around the GTV was created to generate a PTV. The median prescribed dose was 54 Gy (range, 53–55.8 Gy). In terms of the treatment technique, 3D conformal RT planning was performed using a beam eye's view display. Efforts were made to spare the contralateral eye, lens, and optic chiasm. Non-axial beams were used to create a 3D conformal RT plan. The goal was for the 95% line to cover the PTV in its entirety. After treatment, one ONSM showed slight shrinkage and the remaining showed stable findings on repeat MRI. Two patients who could only count fingers prior to treatment had improved visual acuity to 20/70 and 20/200. Five patients noticed clinically significant improvement in visual acuity which was defined as more than three-line improvement on the Snellen chart. Seven patients had stable visual acuity after treatment.

Improvement of color discrimination, contrast sensitivity, and degree of exophthalmos were also observed in several patients.

Patients with ONSM have also been treated with 3DCRT using stereotactic techniques.

Becker et al. (2002) reported the treatment outcomes of 39 patients with primary (n = 15) or secondary (n = 24) ONSM treated with stereotactically guided 3D conformal RT. Conformal and non-coplanar beams were used to deliver 54 Gy in 30 fractions to the tumor. With a median follow-up time of 35.5 months, all patients were alive without evidence of recurrence. Visual fields and visual acuity improved in 6 of 15 and 1 of 16 eyes examined in patients with primary ONSM, respectively. Baumert et al. (2004) reported their results of stereotactic 3D conformal RT for 23 patients with ONSM. All patients received 45–55 Gy in 1.8-Gy fractions using three to five static non-coplanar conformal beams. Micro-MLC or cerrobend blocks were used for beam shaping. The indications for treatment include radiographic or symptomatic progression. At a median follow-up time of 20 months, out of the 22 patients with documented visual decrease prior to treatment, 16 noticed improvement of vision and an additional 5 had no

further progression. Utilizing stereotactic 3D conformal RT, they were able to limit the radiation dose level to the contralateral optic nerve and pituitary gland to < 30% of the prescribed dose. They were also able to spare the optic chiasm and ipsilateral retina in some patients. Landert et al. (2005) treated seven patients with ONSM with stereotactic 3D conformal RT to doses ranging from 50.4 to 54 Gy in 1.8-Gy fractions. Improvement in visual acuity was achieved in 85% of patients. In terms of visual field, 85% had improvement or remained stable. Litre et al. (2007) from France treated eight patients with ONSM with stereotactic 3D conformal RT. The prescribed radiation dose was 45 Gy in 25 fractions. With an average follow-up of 27 months, the tumor control rate was 100%. Vision was re-established in five patients and three patients had improvement of their vision. Diplopia and proptosis resolved in 100% of patients. Vagefi et al. from UCSF reported that among the 35 patients with ONSM treated with stereotactically guided 3D conformal RT, 4 who had neuro-ophthalmologic assessment either during RT or immediately after RT noticed improvement of visual acuity and visual fields signifying a rapid response to RT (Vagefi et al. 2006). The RT dose given ranged from 50 to 54 Gy in

Table 8.1. Summary of treatment results of selected 3D conformal RT series

Series	Number of patients	Technique	Radiation dose (Gy)	Outcomes
Moyer et al. (2000)	1	3D conformal RT	50.4 in 28 fractions	Improved visual acuity and visual field
Turbin et al. (2002)	18	Mixed 2D and 3D conformal RT	40–55 (conventional fractionation)	44.4% showed at least two lines of improvement
Narayan et al. (2003)	14	3D conformal RT	53–55.8 (conventional fractionation)	35.5% had improvement of three lines; 50% had stable vision
Becker et al. (2002)	15	Stereotactic 3D conformal RT	54 in 30 fractions	40% had improvement in vision
Baumert et al. (2004)	23	Stereotactic 3D conformal RT	45–55 (conventional fractionation)	16 of 22 patients with documented visual impairment noticed improvement of vision
Landert et al. (2005)	7	Stereotactic 3D conformal RT	50.4–54 in 1.8-Gy fractions	85% of patients had improved visual acuity and 85% had improved or stable visual field
Litre et al. (2007)	8	Stereotactic 3D conformal RT	45 in 25 fractions	Vision re-established in five and improved in three patients
Vagefi et al. (2006)	4	Stereotactic 3D conformal RT	50–54 (conventional fractionation)	100% had rapid visual improvement

conventional fractionation. The authors suggested RT dose reduction for patients who had rapid response to reduce the risk of complications associated with treatment. Table 8.1 summarizes the treatment results of selected series.

8.4
Treatment Related Toxicity

Acute toxicities are usually mild and manageable and they include fatigue, focal alopecia, skin erythema. Rarely, increased orbital or eye pain can occur. Because of the close proximity of ONSM to critical structures, some amount of radiation will be delivered to those structures even when a conformal technique is used. Efforts should be made to avoid structures such as the contralateral eye, the optic chiasm, the lens of the ipsilateral eye, the pituitary gland, and the ipsilateral lacrimal gland. Late radiation injury to those structures can potentially lead to complications such as visual deficits, cataracts, dryness of eye, or hypopituitarism. Radiation-induced visual deficits can be a result of damage to the optic chiasm (Parsons et al. 1994a), ipsilateral optic nerve (Parsons et al. 1994a), or retina (Parsons et al. 1994b). Hypopituitarism can present as hyposecretion of growth hormone, thyrotropin, corticotrophin, luteinizing hormone, and follicle-stimulating hormone (al-Mefty et al. 1990).

Based on the data in the literature, the most common quoted tolerance doses for a 5% complication in 5 years (TD$_{5/5}$) for various structures are summarized in Table 8.2 (Emami et al. 1991).

Based on the nominal standard dose (NSD) formulation, Goldsmith et al. (1992) analyzed 34 reported patients and 1 from UCSF with radiation-induced optic neuropathy (RON). From those patients, the RON-threshold isotoxicity was determined. An optic ret model was used for the analysis. The analysis suggested that the optic nerve can tolerate 54 Gy in 30 fractions in 1.8-Gy fractions. Details of the model are available to interested readers (Goldsmith et al. 1992).

The typical radiation dose prescribed to ONSM is close to or exceeds the tolerance of these structures. With the use of good 3D conformal RT techniques, the risk of damage to these structures can be significantly decreased. In the study by Turbin et al. (2002), 33% of 18 patients treated with RT alone developed toxicities including retinopathy, persistent iritis, and temporal lobe atrophy. However, some patients were treated with 2D RT. In the study from University of Michigan, the acute toxicities were mild (Narayan et al. 2003). Alo-

Table 8.2. TD 5/5 for critical structures (Emami et al. 1991)

Structure	Dose
Optic nerve	50 Gy
Optic chiasm	50 Gy
Retina	45 Gy
Lens	10 Gy

pecia was the most common complication. One patient (7%) developed corneal inflammation. The late complications were also mild. Out of the 14 patients treated, one developed dryness of the affected eye, 1 developed grade 2 radiation retinopathy but with improved visual acuity, 2 developed iritis that responded to steroid eyedrops, and 1 developed orbital pain that was thought to be related to underlying migraine.

Other studies utilizing stereotactic techniques to deliver 3D conformal RT also yielded low toxicity rates. Becker et al. (2002) did not observe any radiation-induced optic neuropathy or radiation necrosis in the 15 patients with primary ONSM treated with stereotactically guided 3D conformal RT to a dose of 54 Gy in 1.8-Gy fractions. Baumert et al. (2004) reported similar low toxicity rates for the 23 patients treated with stereotactically guided 3D conformal RT for ONSM. In terms of acute effects, one patient (4%) developed eyelid edema, one (4%) had a short term increase of pain, and all had some degree of local alopecia. In terms of late effects, one patient (4%) developed visual deterioration after treatment and one (4%) developed radiation retinitis and vitreous hemorrhage 4 years after treatment. Landert et al. (2005) reported visual deterioration in one (15%) of seven patients with stereotactically guided 3D conformal RT for ONSM. Litre et al. (2007) from France reported no toxicity for the eight patients treated with stereotactically guided 3D conformal RT for ONSM.

References

al-Mefty O, Kersh JE, Routh A, Smith RR (1990) The long-term side effects of radiation therapy for benign brain tumors in adults. J Neurosurg 73:502–512

Baumert BG, Villa S, Studer G, Mirimanoff RO, Davis JB, Landau K, Ducrey N, Arruga J, Lambin P, Pica A (2004) Early improvements in vision after fractionated stereotactic radiotherapy for primary optic nerve sheath meningioma. Radiother Oncol 72:169–174

Becker G, Jeremic B, Pitz S, Buchgeister M, Wilhelm H, Schiefer U, Paulsen F, Zrenner E, Bamberg M (2002) Stereotactic fractionated radiotherapy in patients with optic nerve sheath meningioma. Int J Radiat Oncol Biol Phys 54:1422–1429

Dutton JJ (1992) Optic nerve sheath meningiomas. Surv Ophthalmol 37:167–183

Emami B, Lyman J, Brown A, Coia L, Goitein M, Munzenrider JE, Shank B, Solin LJ, Wesson M (1991) Tolerance of normal tissue to therapeutic irradiation. Int J Radiat Oncol Biol Phys 21:109–122

Eng TY, Albright NW, Kuwahara G, Akazawa CN, Dea D, Chu GL, Hoyt WF, Wara WM, Larson DA (1992) Precision radiation therapy for optic nerve sheath meningiomas. Int J Radiat Oncol Biol Phys 22:1093–1098

Goldsmith BJ, Rosenthal SA, Wara WM, Larson DA (1992) Optic neuropathy after irradiation of meningioma. Radiology 185:71–76

Landert M, Baumert BG, Bosch MM, Lutolf UM, Landau K (2005) The visual impact of fractionated stereotactic conformal radiotherapy on seven eyes with optic nerve sheath meningiomas. J Neuroophthalmol 25:86–91

Lee AG, Woo SY, Miller NR, Safran AB, Grant WH, Butler EB (1996) Improvement in visual function in an eye with a presumed optic nerve sheath meningioma after treatment with three-dimensional conformal radiation therapy. J Neuroophthalmol 16:247–251

Litre CF, Noudel R, Colin P, Sherpereel B, Peruzzi P, Rousseaux P (2007) Fractionated stereotactic radiotherapy for optic nerve sheath meningioma: eight cases (in French). Neurochirurgie 53:333–338

Melian E, Jay WM (2004) Primary radiotherapy for optic nerve sheath meningioma. Semin Ophthalmol 19:130–140

Moyer PD, Golnik KC, Breneman J (2000) Treatment of optic nerve sheath meningioma with three-dimensional conformal radiation. Am J Ophthalmol 129:694–696

Narayan S, Cornblath WT, Sandler HM, Elner V, Hayman JA (2003) Preliminary visual outcomes after three-dimensional conformal radiation therapy for optic nerve sheath meningioma. Int J Radiat Oncol Biol Phys 56:537–543

Parsons JT, Bova FJ, Fitzgerald CR, Mendenhall WM, Million RR (1994a) Radiation optic neuropathy after megavoltage external-beam irradiation: analysis of time-dose factors. Int J Radiat Oncol Biol Phys 30:755–763

Parsons JT, Bova FJ, Fitzgerald CR, Mendenhall WM, Million RR (1994b) Radiation retinopathy after external-beam irradiation: analysis of time-dose factors. Int J Radiat Oncol Biol Phys 30:765–773

Turbin RE, Thompson CR, Kennerdell JS, Cockerham KP, Kupersmith MJ (2002) A long-term visual outcome comparison in patients with optic nerve sheath meningioma managed with observation, surgery, radiotherapy, or surgery and radiotherapy. Ophthalmology 109:890–899; discussion 899–900

Vagefi MR, Larson DA, Horton JC (2006) Optic nerve sheath meningioma: visual improvement during radiation treatment. Am J Ophthalmol 142:343–344

9

Intensity Modulated Radiotherapy for Optic Nerve Sheath Meningioma

Jose Hinojosa, Bin S. Teh, Arnold C. Paulino,
Jorge Omar Hernandez, and E. Brian Butler

CONTENTS

J. Hinojosa, MD
ABC Medical Center, Mexico City, Mexico
c/o The Methodist Hospital, 6565 Fannin, AX121-B, Houston,
TX 77030, USA

J. O. Hernandez, Ph.D
ABC Medical Center, Mexico City, Mexico. c/o The Methodist
Hospital, 6565 Fannin, AX121-B, Houston, TX 77030 USA

B. S. Teh, MD
Radiation Oncology Department, The Methodist Hospital,
6565 Fannin, DB1-077, Houston, TX 77030, USA

A. C. Paulino, MD
Radiation Oncology Department, The Methodist Hospital,
6565 Fannin, DB1-077, Houston, TX 77030, USA

E. B. Butler, MD
Radiation Oncology Department, The Methodist Hospital,
6565 Fannin, DB1-077, Houston, TX 77030 USA

KEY POINTS

Primary optic nerve sheath meningioma is an uncommon anatomical location for meningioma. These patients have a poor visual prognosis without treatment. In recent years, radiotherapy, mainly fractionated stereotactic radiosurgery/radiotherapy (SRS/fSRT), have been successfully utilized and has achieved superior results in stabilizing or improving vision when compared with surgery or observation. On the other hand intensity modulated radiotherapy (IMRT), although currently available in many centers around the world, is a relatively unexplored modality in the treatment of ONSM. IMRT allows an optimized dose distribution to the target while avoiding and/or limiting high radiation doses to the surrounding normal tissues, leading to decreased toxicity. IMRT is an attractive and feasible option for the treatment of ONSM. Prospective studies comparing different radiotherapeutic modalities are required to evaluate outcome and complications, as well as to develop clinical guides to standardize its therapeutic approach.

Introduction

Primary optic nerve sheath meningioma (ONSM) is an uncommon orbital tumor (Eddleman and Liu 2007). It comprises 2% of all tumors in this location and 1%–2% of all meningiomas. Although rare in incidence, the clinical manifestations of the ONSM can affect the quality of life of patients. Despite a very indolent course,

Table 9.1. Radiotherapy modalities

Technique	Description
Fixed field delivery systems	Field size is approximately 5 cm × 5 cm There is no attempt to block normal tissues The patient is treated with opposed fields (right and left lateral fields)
Fixed fields with custom blocks	Field size is again 5 cm × 5 cm The fields are opposed but custom blocks are placed to shield normal tissues from being irradiated
Fractionated stereotactic radiotherapy/radiosurgery or intensity modulated radiotherapy (IMRT)	The radiation oncologist has moved from a shotgun to sniper rifle Small beams are used to create deposition and avoidance patterns The delivery of radiation is more precise and focused The system uses immobilization techniques that guarantee the patient will not move during the course of radiotherapy The immobilization device is typically in the form of a head frame Adjacent critical normal tissues are spared to minimize treatment-related side-effects

the manifestations of ONSM may represent a therapeutic dilemma. The diagnosis of ONSM relies on the clinical presentation and imaging modalities. Magnetic resonance imaging (MRI) with T1-weighted images is the most valuable imaging study and most of the time it obviates the need to biopsy. In some instances, differential diagnoses should be considered especially if patients have a previous history of tumors or malignancies. In general, surgery is a good treatment option for meningioma including ONSM. However, one of the consequences of surgery for optic nerve sheath meningioma is potential visual loss. This makes the treatment with radiation therapy an excellent non invasive option. Reports in the literature have demonstrated the effectiveness of radiation therapy in most series, although involving a small number of patients. Treatment with radiation therapy has gone through technological changes over the last decade. The treatment of ONSM with radiation has evolved from conventional with or without blocks, three-dimensional conformal radiotherapy (3DCRT), to intensity modulated radiation therapy (IMRT), stereotactic radiosurgery/radiotherapy (SRS/SRT) and intensity modulated stereotactic radiotherapy (IMRS). In Table 9.1 we show the different radiotherapy types. Radiotherapy treatment planning has also progressed from using plain X-rays, CT imaging, to the utilization of fusion of the treatment planning CT scans with the diagnostic MRI scans. Strict criteria have been developed for choosing an optimal treatment plan by the radiation oncologist. Verification of the radiation

treatment portal has evolved from weekly plain radiographs and daily positional verification with laser lights to sophisticated image guidance CT scans prior to daily radiotherapy.

9.2
Radiobiological Considerations: Radiation Dose and Fractionation

The α/β ratio is a quantitative measure of sensitivity to changes in dose of radiotherapy delivered per session (fraction size). ONSM is a tumor with a presumed low α/β ratio, therefore a candidate to higher fraction size or a high single dose as in SRS. However, the delivery of single fraction SRS is not always feasible due to the radiosensitive adjacent optic pathway. One of the most important factors in considering radiotherapy for ONSM is the optic pathway. The optic nerves and chiasm are very sensitive to radiation therapy and they are termed in radiobiology as serial late-responding structures. Generally, these serial structures do not have the ability to regenerate like acute-responding tissues, e.g., mucosal membranes. The optic nerves and chiasm are very sensitive to large radiation fraction sizes. The undesired consequence is permanent loss of vision. Doses of radiation in excess of 800 cGy (single fraction, e.g., in SRS) have been documented to show permanent damage to the optic nerve and chiasm. It has also been shown that fraction sizes in excess of 190 cGy may cause increased damage to the optic pathway. Typically, the radiation dose constraint for optic pathway using the fractionated approach is approximately 5040–5400 cGy in 180-cGy fractions. Currently, multiple fractionated radiotheraphy course is preferred to single fraction SRS.

The most utilized ONSM tumor dose is 50.4–54 Gy in daily fractions of 1.8 Gy. The dose per fraction is limited to no higher than 1.9 Gy in order to decrease morbidity related to the adjacent optic pathway. Recent studies (Cozzi et al. 2006) have delivered a wide range of doses ranging from 40 to 59.1 Gy. This could be due to the tumor and patient characteristics (Turbin et al. 2002) such as severity of visual loss, amount of optic atrophy, size of tumor and individual radio-sensitivity. This wide spectrum of radiation doses could also contribute to the difference in the radio-sensitivity and radio-response of the ONSM. As reported by Vagefi et al (2006), some patients showed an early response with visual improvement during the treatment, suggesting that a neuro-ophthalmologic assessment during the radiotherapy course could lead to a customized plan. On the other hand, patients younger than 20 years with a high propensity of more locally aggressive disease and increased rate of recurrences, and patients with intracranial extension and perhaps multifocality (Kim et al. 2005) would probably require a higher than usual radiation dose. Our institution pioneered clinical use of IMRT for CNS tumors in 1994 (Teh et al. 1999). Similarly, we have shown that intensity modulated radiotherapy (IMRT) is safe and efficacious in the primary and adjuvant treatment of intracranial meningioma (Uy et al. 2002) as well as in ONSM (Grant and Cain 1998; Lee et al. 1996; Schroeder et al. 2004) showing excellent results in terms of improved function and treatment outcome.

9.3
Complications

Although radiotherapy is effective for the treatment of ONSM, one needs to be cautious of the treatment-related side-effects because of the proximity of critical radio-sensitive normal tissues such as optic pathway, retina, and brain. The reported (Berman and Miller 2006) acute toxicity included headache, nausea, skin erythema or alopecia. These side-effects were all reversible and usually without long-term sequela. The late toxicity is of major concern and not only related to the intraorbital structures such as optic nerve, chiasm and retina, but also intracranial structures such as pituitary gland and temporal lobe. In the initials report (Cozzi et al. 2006) the complication rate was as high as 33%, mainly related to the old techniques employed. These late radiation-related toxicities included radiation retinopathy, retinal vascular occlusion, persistent iritis and temporal lobe atrophy. The cases of retinopathy (Krishnan et al. 2007) after radiosurgery were related with the total dose to the posterior retina and the proximity of the tumor to the ocular globe.

The tolerance dose (TD) (Kehwar and Sharma 2003; Emami et al. 1991) is a concept which allows us to predict the 5% or 50% of probability of damage to normal tissues in a period of five years, as shown in Table 9.2. This is very important and needs to be respected when delivering the required dose (~50–54 Gy) to control ONSM which is adjacent to the critical radio-sensitive normal tissues. An excellent review (Durkin et al. 2007) of the ophthalmologic complications of radiotherapy has illustrated the numerous important factors involved in its pathogenesis, such as total dose, fraction size, number of fractions and coexisting morbidity. Unfortunately, we do not have the detailed information on

Table 9.2. Tolerance dose 5/5 and 50/5 for the normal tissues involved

Structure	TD 5/5	TD 50/5	Clinical manifestation
Optic nerve	50–55 Gy	60–65 Gy	Optic neuritis
Retina	45–50 Gy	55–60 Gy	Retinopathy
Lens	8–10 Gy	15–18 Gy	Cataract
Ocular surface	35 Gy	50 Gy	Xerophthalmia
Lacrimal gland	30 Gy	45 Gy	Xerophthalmia
Brain	50–60 Gy	> 60 Gy	Brain necrosis

TD = Tolerance dose

partial dose-volume-histogram (DVH) data related to toxicity provided by the current technology used for planning and delivery of radiation (MILANO et al. 2007). Currently, we should continue to keep the basic principles of limiting the tolerance dose of the normal tissues in an attempt to diminish the risk of damage (GLATSTEIN 2001) without affecting our therapeutic objective. The fraction size has been found to contribute to optical neuropathy (DURKIN et al. 2007) and fractions larger than 2 Gy have an incidence of 4% vs 0.3% when 1.8 Gy are utilized. Thus, accurate radiotherapy treatment and delivery techniques are important to achieve both conformal treatment and conformal avoidance leading to improved treatment outcome and quality of life.

9.4
Contraindications to Radiotherapy

Very young children are not good candidates for radiotherapy because of the long term sequelae associated with brain irradiation such as neuron-cognitive deficits and second malignancy. However, we have recently published that IMRT is effective and safe in childhood brain tumors until follow-up without any second malignancies (SCHROEDER et al. 2008; KUPPERSMITH et al. 2000). Other possible contra-indications include recur-

rent tumor in the prior irradiated field and the suspect of a radio-induced or radio-resistant tumor. Generally, the second malignancies risk is very small with 1.35% in 10 years and 1.9% in 20 years, with a calculate risk of 0.04% with doses around 45–50.4 Gy, in children less than 3 years and hypothalamus involvement of 1.6% (STIEBER and MEHTA 2007).

9.5
Intensity Modulated Radiotherapy

Intensity Modulated Radiation Therapy (IMRT) was clinically implemented in the early 1990s. From a conceptual standpoint the radiation oncologist went from using a shotgun to using a sniper rifle. Utilizing IMRT the radiation oncologist could sculpt or paint the deposition of radiation within the volume of the target and could also avoid depositing radiation within the volume of critical radio-sensitive normal structures such as retina and optic chiasm. In simplistic terms, this has been achieved by taking two or three large radiation portals (10 cm × 10 cm) and dividing these portals into multiple small portals (1 cm × 1 cm or 2 cm × 2 cm). These small portals have the capability to turn on or off depending on whether the beam will deposit the radiation. If the small beam will deposit radiation

Table 9.3. IMRT advantages and disadvantages

Advantages	Disadvantages
Great conformality (produce concave isodose surface) that could traduce in lower toxicity	Increased risk of second malignances (more monitor units are used resulting in larger total-body radiation dose and more fields are used with more normal tissue exposed to a lower dose) (HALL 2006)
Sharp-dose gradient (close proximity to an OAR) with less toxicity in normal tissue, for example sparing of parotid glands in head and neck irradiation (BUTLER et al. 1999; AMOSSON et al. 2002, 2003)	Concern of geographical missing due to Organ motion Patient setup uncertainty
Allows for dose escalation potentially increasing local control for example in prostate cancer	Carefully monitoring of patients during the whole course and more strict immobilizations techniques
Dose heterogeneity if desired (higher dose to high risk area inside the PTV) in cases with a region containing a major tumor burden or less oxygenated (hypoxic)	Labor intensive, requires meticulous planning (WOO et al. 2003)
	Expensive compared with conformal treatments (In average 2:1 relationship)
	Uncertainty in the dose calculation model
	Trained and experienced radiation staff

in the target or tumor it will stay open. If the beam will deposit radiation in critical normal structures it will close. Radiation oncology has evolved from using a trial and error method of delivering radiation where the radiation oncologist would rely on experience to tell him where the best beam portals were located or attempt the placement of multiple beam portals and evaluate the deposition and avoidance patterns. IMRT is computer controlled in the sense that the radiation oncologist places defined constraints on a computer program. These constraints limit one from depositing radiation in this particular location (e.g., retina), and it allows one to deposit a defined dose of radiation in the target or tumor. The computer uses complex algorithms, and requires a great deal of computer power to achieve these goals. The computer also assists in the delivery of IMRT. As IMRT has evolved, different delivery systems have evolved all trying to achieve the same goal. Although the development of IMRT started 26 years ago, its clinical application is relatively recent, about 13 years, and is currently available in centers around the world, due in part to the widespread acceptance from radiation oncologists, which has increased rapidly since 2002 (MELL et al. 2005). However, most of the multi-institutional clinical trials involving IMRT to date, have been phase I or II and have addressed only safety and performance issues. Despite the attempt of several institutions to make recommendations regarding the use of IMRT, establishing guidelines for clinical trials, implementation of programs, selections of patients and following a systematic quality assurance program, IMRT is a new technology that must show improvement in clinical outcomes (RANDALL and IBBOTT 2006). In Table 9.3 we summarize some of its main advantages and disadvantages; in Table 9.4 we show the different IMRT types (adapted from IMRT COLLABORATIVE WORKING GROUP 2001).

Optic nerve sheath meningioma is a disease process that benefits from the technology of IMRT. As we have moved from the shotgun to the sniper rifle, we must pay

very close attention and understand the anatomical location of the target and critical structures in detail. We also must make sure that the target does not move or we must understand the movement of the target. Targets in the brain do not move like targets elsewhere in the body that move with respiration. So if we immobilize the patient we have immobilized the target in the head or brain. This immobilization process is critical in achieving the goals of deposition and avoidance. Once deposition and avoidance patterns are achieved there needs to be confirmation by the physics department, and radiographic verification that the patient is being treated as planned.

As previously reported (SCHROEDER et al. 2004) we treated 22 patients with ONSM using IMRT with dynamic arcs via the NOMOS Peacock/Corvus system. The prescribed dose ranged from 49.3 to 50.4 Gy with 1.6–2 Gy per fraction. The mean follow-up was 20 months and we found that 83% of patients receiving IMRT alone achieved subjective visual improvement, 17% subjective stable vision. The objective visual field improvement and stabilization were present in 73% and 27% of patients respectively. Those patients previously operated on showed a lesser rate of improvement and higher rate of stabilization both at 40%. Most patients with acute toxicity had grade 1–2 by RTOG (Radiation Therapy Oncology Group) standards. Only one patient who underwent both surgery and radiotherapy had grade 4 RTOG late toxicity (monocular blindness).

More data are needed from well controlled large multi-center cohorts treated with IMRT. Several important IMRT issues such as local control, marginal recurrences, the risk of second malignancies, and partial volume data will need to be answered. Long term careful follow-up is needed to assess the tumor response, local control, treatment-related toxicity and the management criteria variability (GROUP 2001; TEN HAKEN and LAWRENCE 2006).

IMRT has also been shown to be effective in the treatment of intracranial meningiomas (GRANT and

Table 9.4. IMRT types and conformality

IMRT types	Degree of conformality (Group 2001)
Forward-planned segmental multileaf collimator	3
Inverse-planned segmental multileaf collimator	2–4
Dynamic multileaf collimator	2–4
Tomotherapy	2–4

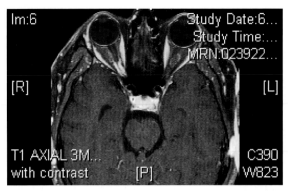

Fig. 9.1. MRI T1 axial 3 mm post fat saturation showing the characteristic "tram track" sign in the right optic nerve sheath

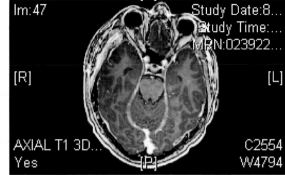

Fig. 9.2. MRI Axial T1 3D with contrast showing reinforcement in the right optic nerve compatible with ONSM

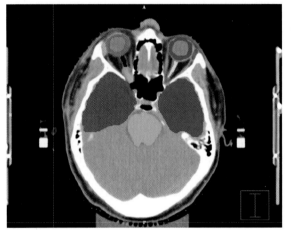

Fig. 9.3. The lesion in the right optic nerve (PTV: planning target volume) (*green*), and the different organs at risk (OAR): right optic nerve (*purple*), left optic nerve (*yellow*), right lacrimal gland (*light pink*) , right temporal lobe (*red*), right orbit (*orange*), eye surface (*blue*), brain stem (*light blue*)

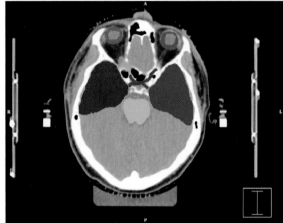

Fig. 9.4. The optic chiasm (*pink*) and its relationship with other OAR as well as the PTV

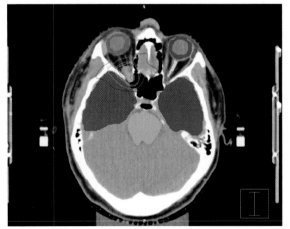

Fig. 9.5. The isodose line distribution: 100% (*red*), 95% (*yellow*), 90% (*green*) and 50% (*blue*)

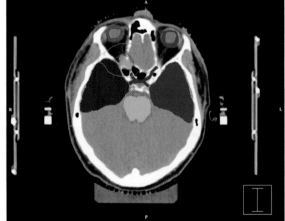

Fig. 9.6. The dose lines close to the optic chiasm: 100% (pink), 95% (blue), 90% (red) and 50% (green)

Cain 1998; Lee et al. 1996; Uy et al. 2002) with an accumulative 5 year local control, relapse free survival and overall survival rates of 91%, 94% and 84% respectively. Effectiveness and safety were also shown for meningiomas located in the skull base and periorbital region challenging locations for both surgery and radiotherapy because of their proximity with organs at risk (OAR) such as optic nerves, optic chiasm, retina, lenses, cranial nerves and brainstem (Milker-Zabel et al. 2007; Pirzkall et al. 2003), with 1–5 years overall survival rates of 98% and 97% respectively with low toxicity rates.

Currently there are no trials directly comparing the best technique (conformal, IMRT or fractionated stereotactic radiosurgery radiotherapy) in irradiating ONSM. There is a preclinical study in small intracranial meningiomas (Fumagalli et al. 2002) evaluating stereotactic radiosurgery using dynamic micromultileaf collimator vs IMRT vs circular collimators. The study concluded that these three modalities are equivalent when lesions have a small volume (around 3 cm³) and spherical shape, just as in the case of ONSM. Another preclinical study (Cozzi et al. 2006) in 12 patients with small benign intracranial tumors (5 of them were meningiomas), which compared Stereotactic Arc Therapy (SRS), IMRT, Helical Tomotherapy (HT), Cyberknife and Intensity-Modulated Multiple Arc Therapy (AMOA), concluded that for PTV coverage the best results were systematically achieved for HT followed by IMRT and AMOA techniques. Meanwhile, for OAR sparing, the best techniques were SRS and Cyberknife for V20 although all the techniques were comparable with AMOA being slightly preferable to IMRT.

Although the treatment of ONSM had changed from conventional and conformal radiotherapy to stereotactic radiosurgery, IMRT (Carrasco and Penne 2004; Jeremic and Pitz 2007; Sitathanee et al. 2006) could be an option, particularly for those facilities without radiosurgery technology available. IMRT, by providing great conformality and sharp-dose gradient, can achieve the goals (Ten Haken and Lawrence 2006) of maximizing target dose, improving target homogeneity and avoiding OAR.

9.5.1
IMRT Procedure

Current recommendations should be followed (IMRT Collaborative Working Group 2001; ICRU 1999):

1. Position – the patient is immobilized and scanned in relocatable frame or mask. The target localization and treatment planning are performed based on CT

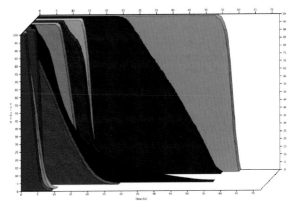

Fig. 9.7. Dose volume histogram: PTV (*green*), right optic nerve (*purple*), left optic nerve (*yellow*), optic chiasm (*pink*), right lacrimal gland (*light pink*), right temporal lobe (*red*), right orbit (*orange*), eye surface (*blue*), brain stem (*light blue*) VH's (images)

scan and MRI (both of them with contrast) fused with planning CT images.

2. Description of volumes – GTV volume was defined as the contrast enhancing lesion (T1 weighted MR images with gadolinium), as shown in Figs. 9.1 and 9.2. The CTV was considered the same as the GTV. The PTV was created by expanding 2–3 mm of the GTV as seen in Figs. 9.3 and 9.4.

3. Dose prescription – 54 Gy in 30 daily fractions of 1.8 Gy to the PTV (95% isodose line). (Fig. 9.5)

4. Mean and maximal doses within PTV and CTV need to be reported. The isodose line distribution is shown in Fig. 9.5.

5. Percentage of PTV and CTV that received the prescribed dose (V 100) need to be reported.

6. Dose constraints – lens < 8–10 Gy, ipsi-lateral and contra-lateral retina < 45 Gy, < 30 Gy for lacrimal gland, Ocular surface < 30 Gy, contra-lateral optic nerve < 50 Gy and optic chiasm < 50 Gy. In Fig. 9.6 the isodose lines can be seen near the optic chiasm and in Fig. 9.7 we evaluated the dose volume histogram (DVH).

References

Amosson CM, Teh BS, Mai WY, Woo SY, Chiu JK, Donovan DT, Parke R, Carpenter LS, Lu HH, Grant WH III, Butler EB (2002) Using technology to decrease xerostomia for head and neck cancer patients treated with radiation therapy. Semin Oncol 29:71–79

Amosson CM, Teh BS, Van TJ, Uy N, Huang E, Mai WY, Frolov A, Woo SY, Chiu JK, Carpenter LS, Lu HH, Grant WH III, Butler EB (2003) Dosimetric predictors of xerostomia for head-and-neck cancer patients treated with the smart (simultaneous modulated accelerated radiation therapy) boost technique. Int J Radiat Oncol Biol Phys 56:136–144

Berman D, Miller NR (2006) New concepts in the management of optic nerve sheath meningiomas. Ann Acad Med Singapore 35:168–174

Butler EB, Teh BS, Grant WH III, Uhl BM, Kuppersmith RB, Chiu JK, Donovan DT, Woo SY (1999) Smart (simultaneous modulated accelerated radiation therapy) boost: a new accelerated fractionation schedule for the treatment of head and neck cancer with intensity modulated radiotherapy. Int J Radiat Oncol Biol Phys 45:21–32

Carrasco JR, Penne RB (2004) Optic nerve sheath meningiomas and advanced treatment options. Curr Opin Ophthalmol 15:406–410

Cozzi L, Clivio A, Bauman G, Cora S, Nicolini G, Pellegrini R, Vanetti E, Yartsev S, Fogliata A (2006) Comparison of advanced irradiation techniques with photons for benign intracranial tumours. Radiother Oncol 80:268–273

Durkin SR, Roos D, Higgs B, Casson RJ, Selva D (2007) Ophthalmic and adnexal complications of radiotherapy. Acta Ophthalmol Scand 85:240–250

Eddleman CS, Liu JK (2007) Optic nerve sheath meningioma: current diagnosis and treatment. Neurosurg Focus 23:E4

Emami B, Lyman J, Brown A, Coia L, Goitein M, Munzenrider JE, Shank B, Solin LJ, Wesson M (1991) Tolerance of normal tissue to therapeutic irradiation. Int J Radiat Oncol Biol Phys 21:109–122

Fumagalli M, Milanesi IM, Fariselli L (2002) Stereotactic radiosurgery using dynamic micromultileaf collimator vs IMRT vs circular collimators for small medium-size intracranial minengiomas. Radiother Oncol 64:S62

Glatstein E (2001) Personal thoughts on normal tissue tolerance, or, what the textbooks don't tell you. Int J Radiat Oncol Biol Phys 51:1185–1189

Grant W III, Cain RB (1998) Intensity modulated conformal therapy for intracranial lesions. Med Dosim 23:237–241

Hall EJ (2006) Intensity-modulated radiation therapy, protons, and the risk of second cancers. Int J Radiat Oncol Biol Phys 65:1–7

ICRU (1999) Prescribing, recording, and reporting photon beam therapy. International Commission on Radiation Units and Measurements. ICRU Rep 62 (Supplement to ICRU Rep 50). ICRU, Bethesda, Maryland 20814 USA

IMRT Collaborative Working Group (2001) Intensity-modulated radiotherapy: current status and issues of interest. Intensity-Modulated Radiation Therapy Collaborative Working Group. Int J Radiat Oncol Biol Phys 51:880–914

Jeremic B, Pitz S (2007) Primary optic nerve sheath meningioma: stereotactic fractionated radiation therapy as an emerging treatment of choice. Cancer 110:714–722

Kehwar TS, Sharma SC (2003) Use of normal tissue tolerance doses into linear quadratic equation to estimate normal tissue complication probability. Radiat Oncol Online J, http://www.rooj.com/Normal%20Tissue%20Comp.htm

Kim JW, Rizzo JF, Lessell S (2005) Controversies in the management of optic nerve sheath meningiomas. Int Ophthalmol Clin 45:15–23

Krishnan R, Kumar I, Kyle G, Husband DJ (2007) Radiation retinopathy after fractionated stereotactic conformal radiotherapy for primary intraorbital optic nerve sheath meningioma. J Neuroophthalmol 27:143–144

Kuppersmith RB, Teh BS, Donovan DT, Mai WY, Chiu JK, Woo SY, Butler EB (2000) The use of intensity modulated radiotherapy for the treatment of extensive and recurrent juvenile angiofibroma. Int J Pediatr Otorhinolaryngol 52:261–268

Lee AG, Woo SY, Miller NR, Safran AB, Grant WH, Butler EB (1996) Improvement in visual function in an eye with a presumed optic nerve sheath meningioma after treatment with three-dimensional conformal radiation therapy. J Neuroophthalmol 16:247–251

Mell LK, Mehrotra AK, Mundt AJ (2005) Intensity-modulated radiation therapy use in the U.S., 2004. Cancer 104:1296–1303

Milano MT, Constine LS, Okunieff P (2007) Normal tissue tolerance dose metrics for radiation therapy of major organs. Semin Radiat Oncol 17:131–140

Milker-Zabel S, Zabel-du Bois A, Huber P, Schlegel W, Debus J (2007) Intensity-modulated radiotherapy for complex-shaped meningioma of the skull base: long-term experience of a single institution. Int J Radiat Oncol Biol Phys 68:858–863

Pirzkall A, Debus J, Haering P, Rhein B, Grosser KH, Hoss A, Wannenmacher M (2003) Intensity modulated radiotherapy (IMRT) for recurrent, residual, or untreated skull-base meningiomas: preliminary clinical experience. Int J Radiat Oncol Biol Phys 55:362–372

Randall ME, Ibbott GS (2006) Intensity-modulated radiation therapy for gynecologic cancers: pitfalls, hazards, and cautions to be considered. Semin Radiat Oncol 16:138–143

Schroeder TM, Yogeswaren ST, Augspurger ME, Lee AG, Teh BS, Lu HH et al. (2004) Intensity modulated radiation therapy for optic nerve sheath meningioma. Int J Radiat Oncol Biol Phys 60 (Suppl 1):S315

Schroeder TM, Chintagumpala M, Okcu MF, Chiu JK, Teh BS, Woo SY, Paulino AC (2008) Intensity-modulated radiation therapy in childhood ependymoma. Int J Radiat Oncol Biol Phys (in press)

Sitathanee C, Dhanachai M, Poonyathalang A, Tuntiyatorn L, Theerapancharoen V (2006) Stereotactic radiation therapy for optic nerve sheath meningioma; an experience at Ramathibodi Hospital. J Med Assoc Thai 89:1665–1669

Stieber VW, Mehta MP (2007) Advances in radiation therapy for brain tumors. Neurol Clin 25:1005–1033, ix

Teh BS, Woo SY, Butler EB (1999) Intensity modulated radiation therapy (IMRT): a new promising technology in radiation oncology. Oncologist 4:433–442

Ten Haken RK, Lawrence TS (2006) The clinical application of intensity-modulated radiation therapy. Semin Radiat Oncol 16:224–231

Turbin RE, Thompson CR, Kennerdell JS, Cockerham KP, Kupersmith MJ (2002) A long-term visual outcome comparison in patients with optic nerve sheath meningioma managed with observation, surgery, radiotherapy, or surgery and radiotherapy. Ophthalmology 109:890–899; discussion 899–900

Uy NW, Woo SY, Teh BS, Mai WY, Carpenter LS, Chiu JK, Lu HH, Gildenberg P, Trask T, Grant WH, Butler EB (2002) Intensity-modulated radiation therapy (IMRT) for meningioma. Int J Radiat Oncol Biol Phys 53:1265–1270

Vagefi MR, Larson DA, Horton JC (2006) Optic nerve sheath meningioma: visual improvement during radiation treatment. Am J Ophthalmol 142:343–344

Woo SY, Grant W III, McGary JE, Teh BS, Butler EB (2003) The evolution of quality assurance for intensity-modulated radiation therapy (IMRT): sequential tomotherapy. Int J Radiat Oncol Biol Phys 56:274–286

Stereotactic Radiation Therapy in Primary Optic Nerve Sheath Meningioma

10

Branislav Jeremić, Maria Werner Wasik, Salvador Villà, Frank Paulsen, Greg Bednarz, Dolors Linero, and Markus Buchgeister

CONTENTS

B. Jeremić, MD, PhD
International Atomic Energy Agency, Wagramer Strasse 5, P.O. Box 100, 1400 Vienna, Austria

M. Werner-Wasik MD
Associate Professor, Residency Program Director, Department of Radiation Oncology, Thomas Jefferson University Hospital, 111 South 11th Street, Philadelphia PA 19107, USA

S. Villà MD, PhD
Department of Radiation Oncology, Hospital Universitari Germans Trias. ICO Badalona, 08916 Badalona. Barcelona, Spain

F. Paulsen, MD
Klinik für Radioonkologie, Universität Tübingen, Hoppe-Seyler-Str. 3, 72076 Tübingen, Germany

G. Bednarz, MD
Department of Radiation Oncology, Thomas Jefferson University Hospital, 111 South 11th Street, Philadelphia, PA 19107, USA

M. Buchgeister, MD
Klinik für Radioonkologie, Universität Tübingen, Hoppe-Seyler-Str. 3, 72076 Tübingen, Germany

KEY POINTS

SFRT is an interesting treatment approach of patients with pONSM which combines advantages of stereotaxy and fractionation. Several institutions used SFRT in patients with progressive visual loss to achieve impressive improvements in both visual fields and visual acuity using relatively modest doses of irradiation (mostly 45–54 Gy, using 1.8- to 2.0-Gy daily fractionation). Excellent visual outcome was almost always accompanied by low toxicity and low tumour reduction on follow-up imaging. Owing to these results, SFRT can be suggested as the new standard treatment approach in patients with pONSM and progressive visual loss.

10.1
Introduction

Stereotactic radiotherapy represents the use of radiation therapy delivered to a stereotactically localized volume of tissue (Leksell 1951, 1971). While the term stereotactic radiosurgery refers to a single-fraction delivery of a high dose of irradiation (Leksell 1971), stereotactic fractionated radiation therapy refers to the use of fractionated irradiation, given once daily, mostly over a period of several weeks. In the last 50 years, various forms of radiation have been used, including gamma rays delivered from multiple cobalt-60 sources using the Gamma-Knife (Arndt 1993), or linear accelerator (Betti et al. 1989), or heavy particles such as helium and protons (Frankel and Phillips 1993; Kjellberg and Preston 1961). In the setting of pONSM, only stereotactic radiosurgery and stereotactic fractionated radiation therapy had been used. They are detailed below.

Stereotactic Radiosurgery

While there are well documented reports on the use of stereotactic, single fraction, radiotherapy (radiosurgery) and occasionally fractionated radiosurgery in various .intracranial meningiomas (KONDZIOLKA et al. 1991, 1999; GIRKIN et al. 1997; LEBER et al. 1998; KLINK et al. 1998; ROSER et al. 2006), only a few of these series included an occasional patient with pONSM (KLINK et al. 1998; KONDZIOLKA et al. 1999; ROSER et al. 2006). One of the possible reasons may include a fear of a high single fraction radiation therapy dose that may lead to toxicity of neighbouring normal tissues. Radiation optic neuropathy was particularly feared complication (TISHLER et al. 1993; GIRKIN et al. 1997; LEBER et al. 1998). In a study of GIRKIN et al. (1997), four patients experienced visual deterioration after 7–30 months after Gamma-Knife radiosurgical treatment. Clinical findings indicated anterior visual pathway involvement. Patterns of field loss included nerve fiber bundle and homonymous hemianopic defects. Gadolinium-enhanced MRI showed swelling and enhancement of the affected portion of the visual apparatus in three patients. In the study of LEBER et al. (1998), a total of 66 sites in the visual system were investigated in 50 patients who had undergone Gamma-Knife radiosurgery for benign skull base tumours. The mean follow-up period was 40 months (range, 24–60 months). Follow-up examinations included clinic/neurological, neuroradiological and neuroophthalmological evaluations. The actuarial incidence of radiation optic neuropathy was zero for patients who received a radiation dose of less than 10 Gy, while it was 26.7% and 77.8% for those who received a dose in the range of 10 to less than 15 Gy and those who received a dose of at least 15 Gy, respectively (p < 0.0001). In contrast to optic pathways (the optic nerve, chiasm, and tract), there was no sign of neuropathy in cranial nerves of the cavernous sinus with the dose received in the range of 5–30 Gy. This study showed that the structures of optic pathways may have higher sensitivity to a single-fraction radiosurgery than other cranial nerves, in particular the oculomotor and trigeminal nerves. These results reconfirmed an earlier experience of the same group (LEBER et al. 1995) who observed that 31% of patients with pre-existing optic neuropathy had their disorders worsen after exposure to radiation doses of 6–16 Gy.

In the case report of a presumed ONSM by KLINK et al. (1998), a patient with pONSM and progressive optic neuropathy and an intact peripheral visual field, stereotactic radiosurgery was delivered using a modified 10-MV linear accelerator by five arcs: two transverse (each 120°), two oblique (each 100°), and one sagittal (100°). Fractionated radiation therapy regimen of 36 Gy in six fractions was used. This dose-fractionation effectively exceeded those traditionally considered as radical (60 Gy in 30 daily fractions (BED values 108 vs 100 Gy). The patient's visual acuity and visual field have remained stable for 2 years following the treatment and the appearance of the tumour did not change by neuroimaging. Mild toxicity was encountered including periorbital oedema, headache and pain, all resolved by 9 months after the stereotactic radiosurgery.

In an interesting report on the use of surgery in pONSM, ROSER et al (2006) reported on three cases of tumour progression after surgical tumour reduction. One patient received stereotactic radiosurgery using Gamma Knife, while two patients were treated using Linear accelerator with 14 Gy prescribed at 60% isodose and 25.6 Gy prescribed at 90% isodose), in order to preserve the opposite nerve. In all cases the treated optic nerve was without function prior to radiation therapy. Neuroradiological follow-up described tumour regression in two cases and a stable disease over 4 years in the other patient. Unfortunately, no further specifications about stereotactic radiosurgery parameters were provided.

Although stereotactic radiosurgery has been used in intracranial meningioma with success, it was extremely rarely used in cases of pONSM. Fear of excessive toxicity high single dose can lead to as well as data showing that this is even more so when once considers optic pathways (versus other intracranial nerves) led to its rare use. In addition, stereotactic fractionated techniques which became widely known and extensively practices in various intracranial tumours, also emerged as successful application in cases of pONSM. While maintaining stereotactic character, their fractionation of the radiation therapy dose was shown to be an advantage in not only high success rate but also low toxicity. It seems, therefore, that stereotactic radiosurgery using a high single-dose of radiation therapy or even several fractions, would not be recommended for future use in patients with pONSM.

Recently, however, ADLER et al. (2006) reported on the use of radiosurgical procedure using novel technological application called the CyberKnife. It is a frameless 6-MV LINAC system for robotic radiosurgery. Radiation is delivered with submillimeter accuracy. As with other forms of stereotaxy, this system presumes a fixed relationship between the target and the skull. Its use eliminates the need for stereotactic frame which has generally been used for a single-fraction radiosurgery Cyber Knife apparatus and was used in 49 consecutive patients with a variety of intracranial tumors, all situated within 2 mm of a "short segment" of the optic apparatus. Of these, 39 patients underwent previous surgery and 6 had previously been treated with conventional fractionated radiation therapy. Cyber Knife delivered two to five sessions to an average tumor volume of 7.7 cm³ and a cumulative average marginal dose of 20.3 Gy. Formal visual testing and clinical examinations were done before treatment and at follow-up intervals beginning at 6 months. After a mean visual field follow-up of 49 months (range, 6–96 months), vision was unchanged post-radiosurgery in 38 patients, improved in 8 (16%), and worse in 3 (6%). In each instance, visual deterioration was accompanied by tumor progression that ultimately resulted in patient death. These results showed that fractionated (multisession) radiosurgery may result in preservation of visual function in patients with perioptic tumors. While there are no data confirming these observations in patients with ONSM, it remains the subject of speculative optimism to consider this technique in selected pONSM. Furthermore, recent report by Romanelli et al. (2007) presented initial data on three patients with pONSM (two intraorbital and one intracanalicullar patient) diagnosed based on neuroimaging only; no biopsy was performed. In all three patients, slow but appreciable impairment in visual functioning was observed. Treatment was instituted with 20 Gy given in 4 fractions being prescribed as an 80% isodose in 4 days. Imaging was repeated every 6 months and thorough neuroophthalmological evaluation was performed every 3 months. While no changes in lesion size was observed over time on serial images, progressive improvement in visual fields and acuity was documented in all three patients. After 1 year, full restoration to normal vision was diagnosed in all patients. Visual fields and acuity restoration have remained stable for 42, 32, and 30 months, respectively, since the irradiation. No information, unfortunately, was provided regarding the side-effects of such treatment, although authors discussed "safety" of their fractionation regimen as opposed to "more aggressive" regimen of 21 Gy delivered in three fractions which have led to loss of vision in one patient in the series of Adler et al. (2006).

10.3
Stereotactic Fractionated Radiation Therapy

Stereotactic fractionated radiation therapy combined advantages of stereotactic approach and biological advantages of fractionating the total tumour dose. While in cases of pONSM, total tumour doses used usually ranged from 45 to 54 Gy, they have unequivocally been given using standard fractionation, e.g. 1.8–1.9 Gy per fraction. Different treatment techniques were used, described in detail below.

10.3.1
Treatment Techniques

10.3.1.1
Thomas Jefferson University, Philadelphia (US) Approach

This part of the chapter summarizes experience of Thomas Jefferson University, Kimmel Cancer Centre, Department of Radiation Oncology with the X-Knife/ Varian 600SR SRS/SRT system and more recently with BrainLab/Novalis SRT systems for optic nerve sheath meningioma. We describe the treatment planning and delivery with multiple isocenter using circular collimators of the X-Knife system and delivery with a single isocenter using the Novalis micro-multileaf collimator.

We commissioned an X-Knife/Varian 600SR 6MV linear accelerator designed for and dedicated to stereotactic radiosurgery and fractionated stereotactic radiotherapy in 1994 (Das et al. 1996) This unit was used from its inception to treat various benign central nervous system tumours, such as acoustic schwannomas, non-acoustic schwannomas, meningiomas (including optic nerve sheet meningiomas, ONSM), pituitary tumours, craniopharyngiomas and others with SRT, using standard daily fractions of 1.8 Gy (rarely, 2.0 Gy). Total doses ranged from 50.4 to 54 Gy.

Patients are referred mostly from the neighbouring Wills Eye Hospital in Philadelphia and the Department of Neurological Surgery of Thomas Jefferson University Hospital. Their cases are presented and discussed at the weekly Stereotactic Tumour Board, attended by the neurosurgeons, radiation oncologists, neuroradiologists, and neurooncologists. Treatment recommendations are given as agreed by all members of the Tumour Board. Most patients with ONSM were diagnosed based on imaging criteria only, although very few had had prior surgical procedures. They were treated with SRT irrespective of the degree of vision preservation on presentation, with only single patients receiving SRS in the blind eye. Pre-treatment evaluation consisted of history and physical examination by the neurological surgeon and radiation oncologist, as well as detailed visual function evaluation by an ophthalmologist, most often a neuroophthalmologist. Patients were followed on a regular basis by the same physicians and underwent

MRI scans of the brain every 6 months, then every 12 months.

Gross Tumour Volume (GTV) was defined on MRI images, fused to the orbital CT scans. GTV comprised the tumour alone and not the entire optic nerve. No margin was added to the GTV to create CTV or PTV. Normal structures which were routinely contoured included the optic nerves, optic chiasm, eye globes and lenses. The maximum allowed dose to the optic chiasm was in the range of 54–57 Gy, depending on the circumstances. Dose Volume Histograms (DVH) were always used to assess the dose distribution to the GTV and normal organs.

10.3.1.1.1
X-Knife-based SRT with Relocatable Frame and Multiple Isocenter Technique

For X-Knife-based SRT, the pre-treatment patient preparation involves the customized design of a lightweight relocatable frame – the Gill-Thomas-Cosman (GTC) frame (KOOY et al. 1994) , which is a large "halo" device that is attached to the patient with custom molded devices that fit into the oral cavity (based on dental impression of patient's upper dentition) and conform to the shape of the occipital region at the back of the head (Fig. 10.1). Day-to-day accuracy of the GTC frame can be verified using a special device called the "depth conformation helmet", a plastic hemispherical shell that allows for the measurement of the distance between the shell and the head surface at a number of locations.

Contrast-enhanced CT data are obtained in the frame with a localization cage attached. The patient is removed from the frame and a gadolinium enhanced MR scan is obtained next. Both imaging datasets are electronically transferred to the treatment planning workstation where they are fused into one composite image for treatment planning purposes. Due to the high spatial fidelity of CT data, the CT dataset is an obligatory imaging dataset for treatment planning. The patient is discharged home and returns for treatment inception usually a week to 10 days later. In the X-Knife system the dose is delivered by using the arc rotation of the linac radiation beam around the linac isocenter. Beam collimation is accomplished using circular collimators (cones) ranging from 0.5 cm to 5 cm in diameter. For single isocenter treatment, the treatment planning relays on selecting the cone size, which covers the target and placing a number of arcs to deliver the radiation dose (Fig. 10.2). For irregular targets multiple cones, each placed at a new isocenter, can be combined to cover the target (Fig. 10.3). Adjusting the placement, lengths and weights of the arcs and the weights of the isocenters, can shape the dose cloud (Fig. 10.4).

Because of the linear shape of ONSM, the X-Knife treatment planning and delivery necessarily involved multiple overlapping isocenters. This created dose inhomogeneity along the axis of the optic nerve. With the advent of the Novalis unit, we have since adopted treatments based on a single isocenter which are much more efficient and which yield much higher dose homogeneity along the axis of the optic nerve with dynamic arc technique.

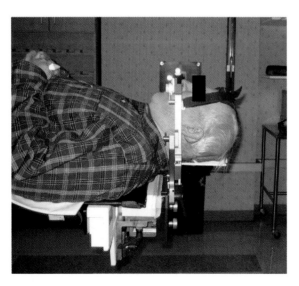

Fig. 10.1. The Gill-Thomas-Cosman relocatable frame

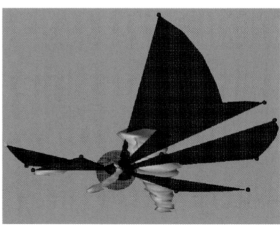

Fig. 10.2. X-Knife treatment with single collimator and multiple arcs of various lengths and orientations

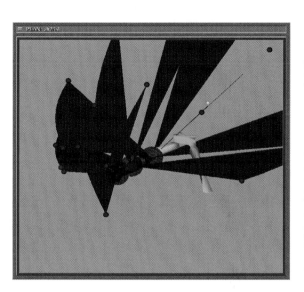

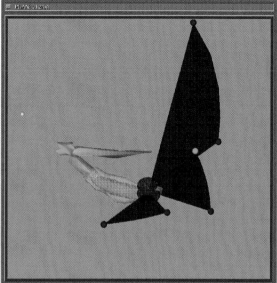

Fig. 10.3. For irregular targets, such as ONSM, multiple cones, each placed at a new isocenter, can be combined to cover the target

Fig. 10.4. X-Knife treatment with multiple isocenters for ONSM. The dose cloud is shaped by adjusting the isocenters weight and arcs lengths, placements and weights

10.3.1.1.2
The BrainLab/Novalis SRT System with Mini-multileaf Collimator

Patients can be treated on the Novalis system either using the GTC frame or a multi-component thermoplastic head mask (BrainLab, Germany), which is custom-fitted to the shape of the patient's head (GEORG et al. 2006). The mask consists of one posterior shell and two anterior components. In addition to the two anterior parts, a special nose bridge is molded from thermoplastic beads to minimize head rotation during repositioning. All components are mounted on a U-shaped metal frame and locked together with a set of plastic clips with adjustable spacers to allow for the mask shrinkage (Fig. 10.5a). The Novalis treatment-planning workstation provides a number of planning options ranging from dynamic arc treatment, to conformal static arcs or

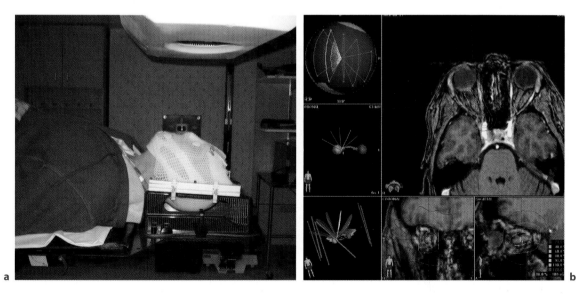

Fig. 10.5a,b. BrainLab's thermoplastic head mask (**a**) and isodose distribution in ONSM patient (**b**)

stereotactic IMRT (Solberg et al. 2001). At our institution, most treatment plans involve a single isocenter treatment with five non-coplanar arcs utilizing the dynamic arc method. With micro-multileaf collimation, this technique allows for both high target conformality and high dose homogeneity (Fig. 10.5b).

We published our initial results of SRT for ONSM involving 33 optic nerves in 30 patients in 2002 (Andrews et al. 2002). The median prescription dose was 51 Gy (range: 50.4–54 Gy) and the median follow-up, 21 months. Of 22 optic nerves with vision before SRT, 20 nerves (92%) demonstrated preserved vision and 42% manifested improvement in visual acuity and/or visual fields. Four patients (13%) had post-treatment morbidities, including visual loss (two patients), optic neuritis (one patient) and transient orbital pain (one patient). At the time of publication, no tumour progression was reported on MRI scans. Six patients were monitored with ^{111}In-octreotide scintigraphy which demonstrated significant metabolic responses following SRT.

Most recently, we updated our experience (up to 2006) to include a total of 50 patients with ONSM (manuscript in preparation). Follow-up data were available for 38 patients (one treated to both eyes), with 12 lost to follow up. Five patients had no light perception in the involved eye on presentation (one lost to FU). Among the remaining 34 patients with vision on presentation, 20 (59%) experienced improvement in visual acuity and/or visual fields and 11 (32%) had stable vision, for a total of 31/34 (91%) preserving vision. Three patients (9%) had worse vision, in one case attributed to tumour progression. One of the two remaining received SRT with the BrainLab system.

Two cases below illustrate an improvement in visual fields (Fig. 10.6) and an early visual acuity improvement, occurring during the SRT course and within 3 months from SRT completion (Fig. 10.7). Such an early effect is not rare and it is difficult to explain biologically.

Date and SRT Dose	R eye visual acuity
6-23-05 consultation	20/50
7-13-05 10.8 Gy	20/200
7-20-05 19.8 Gy	20/50
7-27-05 28.8 Gy	20/70
8-3-05 37.8 Gy	20/30
11-22-05 FU 3 months	20/20

Fig. 10.7. Early improvement in visual acuity in a patient with right ONSM treated with SRT

10.3.1.2
BrainLAB Technique (Barcelona, Spain)

Since 2000 this technique has been available at departments of Radiation Oncology of Centro Médico Teknon-CMT, and Catalan Institute of Oncology-ICO, both in Barcelona, Spain.

Radiation therapy planning was done in several phases:

1. Immobilization with triple thermoplastic mask (Figs. 10.8a,b–10.11a,b). Material for positioning is composed by head resting-place that includes head-rest, mask ring, screws for fixing vertical posts and cam locks to put into cube for checking coordinates. The non-invasive triple mask (top, rear, and middle mask) enables precise and easy repeatable patient fixation. The mask of thermo-transformable material is individually moulded for each patient and secured to the mask ring (BrainLAB 2000; Villà et al. 2000; Brell et al. 2006). Mask should be heated in water to 70–80 °C. Different steps are needed to mould the entire mask. Patient's head is left and snap the mask onto the upper side of the vertical posts and put down onto the headrest. In approximately 1 min mask material is hardening. After that, middle mask is placed in the centre of the middle's face, carefully stretched. A T-shaped form nose bridge mould is added to the middle mask using rolled loose pellets after heating to optimize head fixation. The next step is to place the top mask centrally over the patient's face ensuring that the curve in the mask is placed towards the patient's mouth, but does not cover it. Top mask is secured by clips. Different clips and

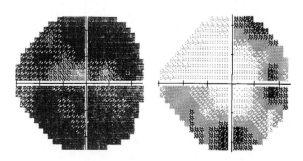

Fig. 10.6. Humphrey automated perimetry (24-2 central threshold) of left visual field in patient with left ONSM at pretreatment (*left*) and at 11 months after SRT (*right*)

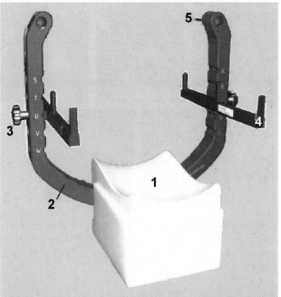

a

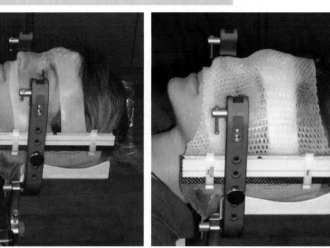

b

Fig. 10.8a,b. Immobilization system – material for positioning and head fixation.
a Head resting-place: 1 – headrest, 2 – mask ring, 3 – screws, 4 – vertical posts, 5 – cam locks.
b Mask system. Courtesy of BrainLAB, Heimstetten, Germany

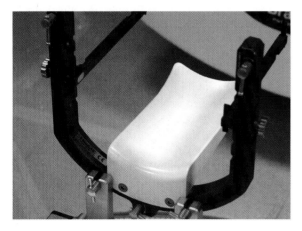

Fig. 10.9. Head resting-place at time of treatment at coach position before starting RT session

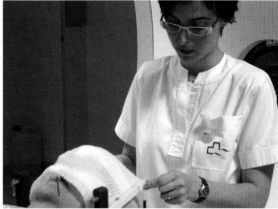

Fig. 10.10. Head fixation using a triple thermo-plastic mask at time of treatment. *Arrow* shows an additional dental support strip for superior maxillary fixation

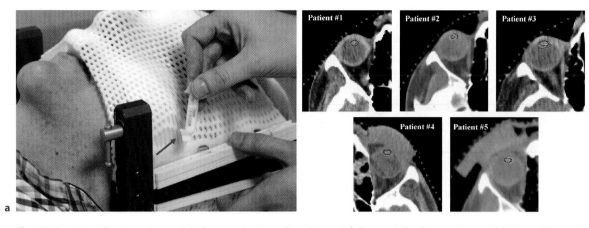

a   b

Fig. 10.11. a Head fixation using a triple thermo-plastic mask at time of treatment. *Arrow* shows a plastic clip (with five different thickness from 0 mm to 4 mm). It permits a comfortable positioning for every patient regarding change of weigh (for corticosteroids or malnutrition). No errors in precision are detected. **b** Lenses defined on each control CT scan (drawn in different colours) and the respective lenses defined on the planning CT after CT-to-CT skull registration (MIRALBELL et al. 2007)

spacers are needed to adapt size and head anatomy for every patient and fix rear mask to top mask. An additional dental support strip for superior maxillary fixation is added to improve its quality.

Position of ocular balls. Eyes should be closed for simulation and treatment. Patients are required to close gently both eyes on MRI scan and on CT scan, and for every session thereafter. With this simple movement, we reported that margins of 3 mm around the target may be necessary to safely treat these tumours under ideal set-up conditions. Experience from ocular melanoma was translated to ONSM (MIRALBELL et al. 2007). As can be seen in Fig. 10.11, lenses for ipsilateral affected eye was used to be defined on each control CT scan and the respective lenses defined on the planning CT after CT-to-CT skull registration.

2. Co-registration of CT and MRI. After cranial immobilization, all patients underwent a planning CT scan with fiducial rods attached to the head frame. CT images are obtained from the scalp vertex through the brain using 2–3 mm thick slices (acquisition time is of 30–40 s) and transferred to the treatment planning system (TPS), BrainScan 5.1 (BrainLAB A.G., Heimstetten, Germany). Contrast for CT is used in some cases. CT to MRI registration is performed for each patient by automatic alignment of bone structures on the two image sets. Target volumes and organs at risk (OARs) are defined on the MR images

and projected on to the respective CT sets. CT scans are used for dosimetric calculations.

Definition of target volumes (GTV=CTV, and PTV) could be done in any of images (only CT scan volume definition is very useful in some patients; see Fig. 10.12). GTV and CTV are defined as the whole optic nerve due to the difficulty to separate tumour itself of the rest of nerve in many cases. PTV is defined with a margin of 3 mm (MIRALBELL et al. 2007). As a rule, all the following OARS have to be defined: retina, contra-lateral optic nerve, chiasm, lens, brain-stem, lachrymal gland, and pituitary.

3. Dosimetry. Any of the facilities from TPS could be used such as conventional circular arc radiosurgery (RS), dynamic arc RS, conformal RS using multiple static shaped beams (Fig. 10.13), and IMRS implemented by either static or dynamic micro multi-leaf collimator (mMLC) techniques (Fig. 10.14). The so-called m3 mMLC "moulds" target shape in any angle and field (beam eye view).

4. Dose. Prescribed total dose ranges between 50 and 54 Gy at ICRU point, 25–30 fractions, 1.8–2 Gy per fraction, once a day (Fig. 10.15).

5. OARS. Contra-lateral optic nerve, chiasm, lens, lachrymal gland, pituitary, brain-stem, and retina are systematically drawn (Fig. 10.15).Optimal organ dose constraints are as follows: retina: 50 Gy; lens: 9 Gy; optic nerve and chiasm: 55 Gy; lacrymal gland: 30 Gy

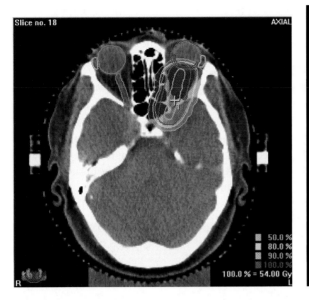

Fig. 10.12. Isodoses distribution on the PTV. The patient was planned using the CT scan

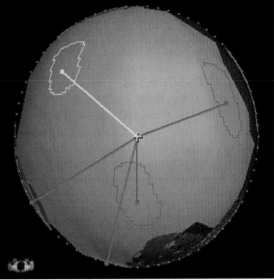

Fig. 10.13. In this figure it can be seen an example of five fix fields conformed by micromultileaf m3 collimator. The collision map to guarantee no accidents at the treatment set up can also be observed

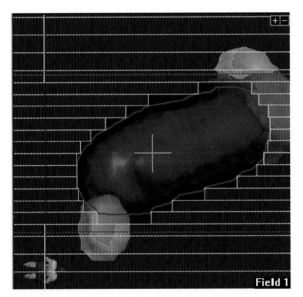

Fig. 10.14. Image of the m3 micromultileaf collimator (beam eye view)

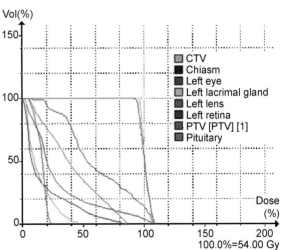

Fig. 10.15. Dose Volume Histogram (DVH) for GTV and PTV, and most relevant organs at risk for the specific case

Dose Volume Histogram (DVH) must always be done and displayed for GTV, CTV and PTV, and for most relevant organs at risk for every specific case (Fig. 10.15).

Treatment was performed using a radiosurgery-dedicated 6-MV X-ray beam linear accelerator with a built-in m3 mMLC (Figs. 10.14 and 10.16) (Novalis®, BrainLAB, Heimstetten, Germany). It was installed at Centro Médico Teknon in Barcelona in 2000. This treatment system is able to operate in several modalities (see above). For treatment set-up a cube for checking coordinates is used every fraction to assure minimal isocenter error and good quality assurance (Fig. 10.17). This cube enables one to check the origin of the coordinates (coordinates 0,0,0) at the beginning of set-up and to move to the PTV coordinates.

Three different laser projections (two laterals and one superior-saggital) are projected on coordinates cube and on patient mask (Figs. 10.18 and 10.19). In relation to final dosimetry, different coach and gantry angles are needed to accomplish treatment agreed between physicians and physicists. Coach position must be checked inside the bunker (Fig. 10.16).

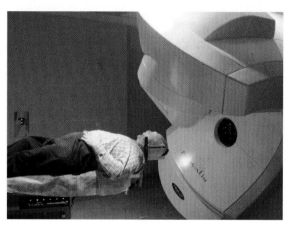

Fig. 10.16. In relation to final dosimetry, different coach and gantry angles are needed to accomplish treatment agreed between physicians and physicists. Treatment position. Table and gantry rotation for a specific treatment field

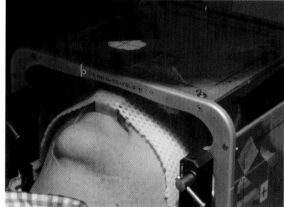

Fig. 10.17. Cube for checking the origin coordinates (coordinates 0,0,0) and the PTV coordinates (*arrow*)

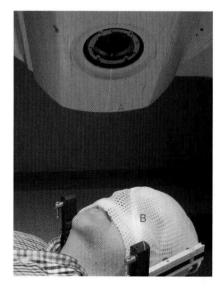

Fig. 10.18. Triple room lasers for checking patient position: lateral laser (**A**) and superior (saggital) laser (**B**)

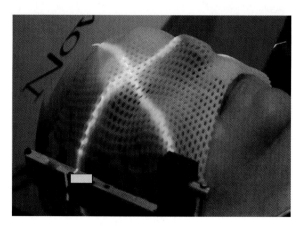

Fig. 10.19. Triple room lasers for checking patient position. Simulation of the isocenter on the centre of the orbit

10.3.1.3
University of Tuebingen, Germany Approach

At Tuebingen, conformal radiotherapy of optic nerve sheath meningioma has been performed with 6-MV photons and a conventional fractionation scheme at a linear accelerator (LINAC) employing a non-invasive rigid mask immobilisation system designed at the German Cancer Research Center, Heidelberg, since 1993 (SCHLEGEL et al. 1992; BECKER et al. 2002a). Treatment planning precedes an interdisciplinary board discussing the indication and target extension for treatment. The target volume comprises the gross visible optic nerve sheath tumour. If this is not clearly distinguishable, the whole optic nerve (GTV) covering the anatomical region of ophthalmological functional deficits, enlarged by necessary safety margins of the used mask immobilisation system represents the planning target volume (PTV). Organs at risk (OARs) in close vicinity such as chiasm, optical nerve, eye globes, lenses, brain stem or the brain itself are segmented in the planning computed tomography (CT) slices. The treatment planning is performed with a commercial planning system (Helax TMS) employing non-coplanar, wedged and individually shaped small treatment portals. A fractionation of 5×1.8 Gy/week up to 54 Gy is used. The immobilisation of the patient to treat this vulnerable region has to be optimised for the correct daily beam application. Several principles can be used to achieve this goal. A relatively simple method is the usage of a rigid mask system with well known immobilisation errors that are taken into account in the definition of the PTV. The individual set-up control is described below. More advanced im-mobilisation systems deal with the whole treatment unit including a visualisation tool (CT) at the LINAC and a robotic table also being able to compensate for rotational errors.

For the approach described in the following section, a rigid relocatable immobilisation mask system with a mean accuracy of 0.8 ± 0.6 mm is used. In an analysis of our first patients 95% of all absolute measures were less than 2.8 mm for transition to the LINAC and 4.6 mm during treatment (KORTMANN et al. 1999). The isocenter setup is performed with a stereotactic localization system described in BECKER et al. (2002a) using stereotactic coordinates. Stereotactic coordinates are used for the transfer of the isocenter to the patient within the immobilisation mask. The process of treatment planning starts with the building of the special removable immobilisation mask system. The mask is made of cast material. For its creation the patient lies supine on a treatment couch with his head resting in an extension made of two curved wooden plates around which the cast material is rolled (Fig. 10.20). The extension is necessary to avoid dosimetric disturbances due to the treatment couch for posterior entry portals or collision between gantry and couch. This enables a wide range of non-coplanar beams. After hardening of the material (about 30–45 min) the mask is cut from chin to above the ear region to allow the patient to leave and re-enter the mask (Fig. 10.21) with reasonable comfort. For planning and treatment the mask is closed with simple fixation locks at each side. The patient holds an emergency trip wire to be able to release the mask fixation locking (Fig. 10.20).

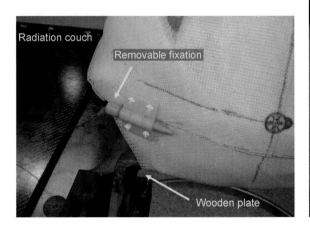

Fig. 10.20. Mask made of casting material rolled around wooden plates, removable fixation for the patients' emergency exit

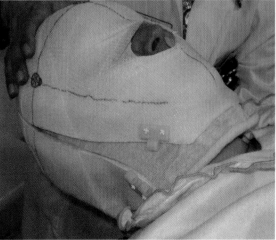

Fig. 10.21. Jaw of the mask and patients' entrance into the mask

During treatment planning a diagnostic MRI and the planning CT are fused (e.g. by mutual information algorithms) in the radiation treatment planning system (RTP) and checked by an experienced radiation oncologist. A stereotactic localisator, that is mounted over the fixation mask (Fig. 10.22) defines the stereotactic coordinate system for the patients' anatomy inside the mask. The planning CT includes the whole head from the top of the scull to the neck to allow for the planning of non-coplanar treatment beams and to estimate the beam direction inside the body (Fig. 10.23). The slice thickness is in the range of 2–3 mm in the region of the PTV to get adequate resolution of the different small sized organs. As the planning CT and a high resolution MRI is co-registered for target volume definition, a contrast media enhanced planning CT is not also necessary. Second, due to the rigid mask system, there is a higher risk for severe complications in case of allergic reactions to the contrast media when such a CT is taken. After co-registration of the planning CT and the MRI, target volumes (GTV, organs at risk) are delineated. The PTV is generated by adding 5 mm to the GTV for the treatment plan that is used for the first 28 fractions up to 50.4 Gy (Fig. 10.24). For the boost of an additional 3.6 Gy, the PTV is reduced by adding only 2 mm safety margin around the GTV.

Optimal beam angles are determined during the radiation treatment planning process with the help of the beams' eye view function of the RTP. The treatment plan is iteratively optimized to achieve a dose distribution according to the guidelines defined by the ICRU 50 report. PTV and OARs define the geometry of each field such that 95% of the prescribed dose surrounds the PTV. An experienced treatment planning team usually achieves a homogeneous dose distribution for the PTV. The dose to brain stem, chiasm or optical nerves should not exceed 54–55 Gy in 1.8-Gy fractions, the dose to the other OARs being as described above in this chapter. Usually 5–6 wedged fields are used. The position of the isocenter for treatment is defined within the stereotactic localisator at the CT. Three translations are given to move the patient from the stereotactic coordinate $(0;0;0)$ to the coordinates of the isocenter $(X;Y;Z)$ (Fig. 10.25) at the set-up for treatment. The z-coordinate is defined by the distance "A" of the metal markers at the surface of the stereotactic localisation tool (Figs. 10.22 and 10.25). Two orthogonal verification beams of standardized field size of 8×8 cm^2 are created and digital reconstructed radiographs (DRR) are printed for following setup verifications at the LINAC. Individualized shielding is achieved by usage of conventional shielding blocks made of MCP96. Every shielding block is controlled before treatment by comparison of the block's light field shape at the LINAC with the scaled beam's outline printed on paper (Fig. 10.26). The deviation of the resulting field has to be in a clinical acceptable range

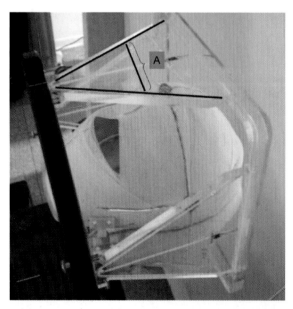

Fig. 10.22. Planning stereotactic localisation tool mounted over the mask; diagonal radiopaque lines with defined distance "A"

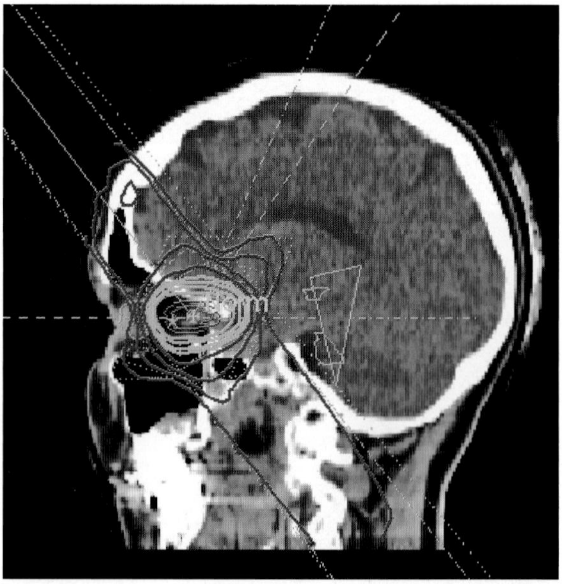

Fig. 10.23. Isodose distribution in a sagittal reconstruction estimating the bodies distribution

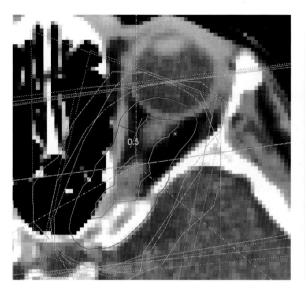

Fig. 10.24. Macroscopic tumour (GTV) of the left optic nerve and 0.5 cm safety margin defining the planning target volume (PTV) up to 50.4 Gy

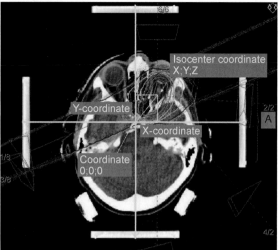

Fig. 10.25. Isodose distribution and translation from the stereotactic origin (0;0;0) to the treatment isocenter (X;Y;Z); distance "A" of the stereotactic localisation tool (see Fig. 10.3)

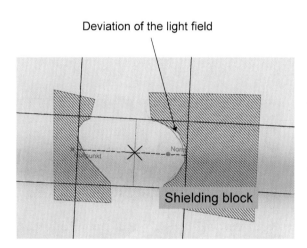

Fig. 10.26. Deviation of the beams light field projected on the shielding block print of the planning system

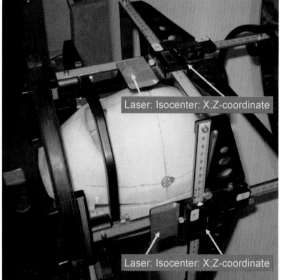

Fig. 10.27. Stereotactic positioning system for the translation of the planning isocenter to the LINAC: (X;Y;Z)-coordinates are set at the displays of the localisator lines and being marked on the mask

depending on the anatomical regions of the deviation of less than 1.5 mm at the isocenter.

The radiation treatment isocenter is transferred to the patient with the aid of a special external stereotactic positioning device (Fig. 10.27). The isocenter lasers' positions are marked on the surface of the mask. The

above-mentioned two orthogonal verification fields are produced and compared with the corresponding planning DRRs (Fig. 10.28). Additionally, the isocenter is controlled by another CT, where the isocenter laser positions marking the set-up position at the LINAC are indicated by soldering wires. The in this way indicated

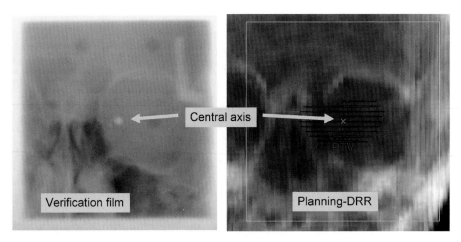

Fig. 10.28. Control of the isocenter by comparison of marked central axis on a verification film with the corresponding DRR of the planning system

treatment isocenter is compared to the one of the corresponding planning CT and corrections are computed for set-up at the LINAC if necessary (Fig. 10.29). After correction of the isocenter, treatment portals are marked at the mask (Fig. 10.30). Analysis of verification films of the isocenter during the first week is used to determine the resulting systematic error which has to be corrected. Weekly isocenter checks follow in the remaining time of treatment.

The planning process is time consuming with respect to the creation of the mask and the planning process at the radiation treatment planning system. Each fraction is in the range of a multiple field irradiation, about 15–20 min. In general the treatment is well tolerated by the patients. A detailed analysis of the first patients has been published (BECKER et al. 2002a; PITZ et al. 2002). This treatment approach can easily be introduced into clinical routine with a fixed protocol of handling. High precision in the daily delivery, an experienced treatment planning team and an interdisciplinary care between neuroophthalmologist, neuroradiologist, neurosurgeon and radiation oncologist are the main characteristics.

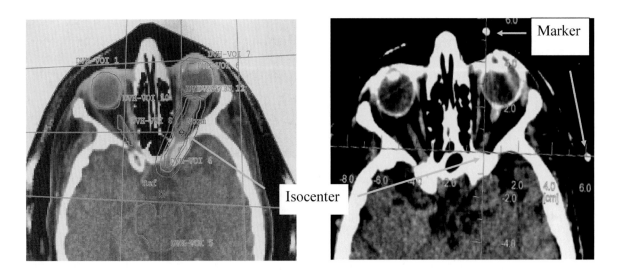

CT planning   CT control

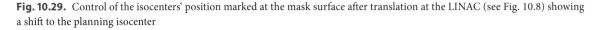

Fig. 10.29. Control of the isocenters' position marked at the mask surface after translation at the LINAC (see Fig. 10.8) showing a shift to the planning isocenter

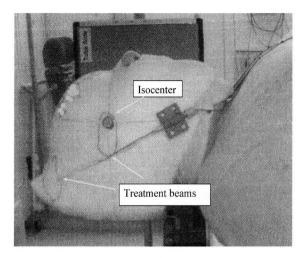

Fig. 10.30. Treatment beams and isocenter marked at the mask surface

10.3.2
Clinical Results

With the introduction of stereotactic principles in radiation oncology, pONSM became one of the major targets, in spite of their relative infrequency. Several institutions used this technique, using protracted, fractionated RT regimens to deliver tumour doses deemed as appropriate for controlling these tumours. While it was earlier recognized that tumour shrinkage was not the main goal of the SFRT, as well as that modest doses (50–55 Gy) are sufficient to produce long-lasting stabilization or improvement of functioning of affected eyes, SFRT as used in pONSM was first introduced and then increasingly practiced in the 1990s. Unfortunately, due to rarity of these tumours, relative sophistication of the techniques used and lack of specific recommendations about the preferred patient group suitable for RT as well as the timing of the use of RT itself, only a few institutions actually provided data for the readerships of major medical/scientific journals.

In the year 2002, we have witnessed a total of four reports coming from three institutions (LIU et al. 2002; ANDREWS et al. 2002; BECKER et al. 2002a; PITZ et al. 2002) which included precise data on treatment planning and delivery of RT. Prolonged follow-up periods were offered as well, all giving better perspective on the use of SFRT in pONSM. In the study of LIU et al. (2002), a total of five patients (three women and two men), ranging in age from 40 to 73 years, presented with progressive visual loss with decreased visual field, visual acuity, and colour vision affecting six eyes (involvement of both optic nerves in one patient). One of these five

patients also presented with proptosis and diplopia. Five eyes had residual vision (range, 20/20 to 20/40), and one eye was completely blind. All five patients were diagnosed clinically and radiographically to have an ONSM. Three were intraorbital, one was intracanalicular as well as intraorbital, and one was left ONSM extending through the optic foramen into the intracranial space and involving the right optic nerve. A patient with an intracranial and bilateral involvement of tumour in both optic nerves initially refused craniotomy and favoured SFRT only to the functioning right optic nerve. The five functional eyes were treated with SFRT using daily dose of 1.8 Gy to a total dose of 45–54 Gy. Gill-Thomas-Cosman head frame (Radionics, Burlington, MA) and the X-knife radiosurgery unit (Radionics) were used. The treatments were planned to encompass the tumour at the 90% isodose line. Patients were followed-up over 1–7 years and diagnostic tests included serial MRI and neuro-ophthalmological examinations done regularly at 3-month intervals. Within 3 months after SFRT, four of the five patients experienced dramatic improvement in visual function. Visual field deficits resolved in all four, visual acuity improved in three, and colour vision improved in two patients. Of the four patients whose visual fields deficits resolved, one patient had resolution of optocilliary shunt vessels. Optic nerve atrophy and optic disc swelling remained unchanged. The fifth patient had stabilization of all visual tests. There was no clinical or radiographic evidence of radiation necrosis or radiation-induced optic neuropathy. According to serial CT and MRI scans, the size of the tumours in all five patients remained unchanged from the time an initial imaging was done.

ANDREWS et al. (2002) provided an analysis on 30 patients (18 women and 12 men; age range 20–75 years) and 33 optic nerves with ONSMs, including three patients with bilateral ONSMs. Nine (29%) of the ONSMs were localized to the intraorbital portion of the optic nerve, 12 (36%) extended to the optic canal and 1 (3%) extended beyond the optic canal to the chiasm. Six ONSMs (18%) involved the optic canals and the chiasm, whereas bilateral ONSM in one patient (3%) involved the entire optic apparatus. In addition, two (9%) cases include involvement of the optic canal and the middle, anterior, and/or posterior fossa. Each patient had experienced significant visual loss and acuity deficits before radiation therapy. All 33 optic nerves had objective signs associated with ONSM. Nine optic nerves were not useful, with either no light perception or light perception only, while the remaining 24 optic nerves were viable and provided useful vision. Then initial diagnosis was made based on either surgical procedure or on the basis of characteristic appearance on T1-weighted contrast-enhanced fat-suppression MRI. A dedicated linear accelerator was designed for radiosurgery and was used in all cases. Gill-Thomas-Cosman relocatable frame was used as well as X-knife 3D treatment planning from Radionics. An average of three isocentres were used and high-conformality was established by noncoplanar beam shaping and differential beam weighting. A total dose of 50.4 Gy was planned to be delivered in 28 daily fractions of 1.8 Gy delivered in a 5-week period. Pre- and post-SFRT serial clinical and radiographic evaluations, including MRI scans and functional ^{111}In-octreotide single-photon emission computed tomographic (SPECT) scintigraphy were compared to establish objective tumour response. Patients were examined during the first 3 months after SFRT and every 6 months thereafter. Median clinical follow-up time was 89 weeks (range, 9–284 weeks). The median number of fractions administered was 28.5, the median isosurface dose was 51 Gy (range 50.4–54.0 Gy), and the median number of isocentres was 3. Of 24 optic nerves with useful vision before SFRT, 22 (92%) demonstrated either stability (n = 12; 50%) or improvement (n = 10; 42%) in visual acuity and fields at follow-up. Tumour volume reduction was observed in four (13%) patients, with no evidence of tumour progression or recurrence in all patients. Four (13%) patients experienced treatment related toxicity, including two (6%) patients with visual loss, one (3%) patient experiencing optic neuritis and one (3%) patient experiencing transient orbital pain.

Becker et al. (2002a) reported on their experience with a total of 39 patients with either primary (n = 15) or secondary (n = 24) patients with ONSM treated between 1994 and 2000. All patients with primary ONSM and 18 patients with secondary ONSM were irradiated after disease progression as determined by imaging and/or ophthalmologic testing. An individually formed, removable, and relocatable mask, consisting of cast material was used to immobilize the patient's head and neck, while being attached to the stereotactic base frame. VOXEL-Plan-Heidelberg and HELAXTMS systems were used for treatment planning purpose. Conformation of the therapeutic radiation dose was done by two to six noncoplanar and individually shaped fields (median, four fields) for primary ONSM. The SFRT dose was 50.40 Gy in 26 daily fractions prescribed to the ICRU reference point with a safety margin of 5 mm. The boost of 3.60 Gy in two fractions was added with a margin of 2 mm. Patients were followed at regular intervals using ophthalmologic and radiooncologic evaluations as well as MRI at 3-month intervals during the first year after SFRT, and at 3- to 6-months intervals during the second year. Endocrinologic testing was performed at 6-month intervals. After the second year of follow-up, the oph-

thalmologic, radio-oncologic, and MRI examinations were done every 6 months and the endocrinologic examinations were performed yearly, unless otherwise indicated by signs/symptoms of the disease. After the end of fifth year, patients were followed annually, with the aforementioned tests used regularly. Follow up ranged from 10 to 73 months for primary ONSM (median, 39 months) and from 10 to 56 months for secondary ONSM (median, 32.5 months). A response to treatment was observed in all 39 patients with ONSM. All patients experienced stable disease (no change) on CT/MRI, and only one patient experienced tumour shrinkage, considered a partial response. All patients were alive at the time of the report without the disease progression. In one patient with primary ONSM, functional deterioration of the contralateral eye occurring 42 months post-SFRT led to verification with MRI, which was inconclusive. Its findings suggested a possibility of either ONSM in the contralateral eye or local recurrence in the treated eye subsequently extending to the other side. Surgery was done and pathologic examination revealed a soft-tissue mass with existing infiltration of lymphocyte and plasma cells. The immunohistochemical finding excluded ONSM and was interpreted as a chronic inflammation. When treatment and isodose charts were evaluated, it was found that this area received only a scattering dose.

Detailed functional outcome analysis on the same group of 15 patients with primary ONSM was provided by Pitz et al. (2002). Ophthalmological investigation included best corrected visual acuity tested with a Snellen chart (Duke-Elder and Smith 1962) at 5-m distance, assessment of a relative afferent papillary defect (RAPD), motility testing, slit lamp investigation of the anterior segment, and funduscopy. Testing of visual fields was done with the Goldman perimeter, and within the 30° area with the Tuebingen manual perimeter or Tuebingen automated perimeter, respectively. To obtain reliable results on follow-up, only similar performance measurements recorded were considered, and only absolute scotomas were evaluated. The evaluation of visual fields was done using a modified Esterman grid (Esterman 1968), indicating the percentage of visual field loss by counting the number of absolute defects. After a mean follow-up of >3 years, none of the seeing eyes treated suffered from deterioration of visual function. An increase in visual acuity of two or more lines was found in one patient; amelioration of visual field defects of at least 8% was noted in five patients; one patient experienced rather dramatic improvement in the better eye from 72% visual loss to 4%. Stable disease was observed in eight patients. However, three of these patients were already blind or nearly blind at SFRT initiation. Thus, the functional improvement was obtained in 7 out of 15 (46%) patients, and 7 out of 16 (43%) eyes (including the better eye of patient with bilateral involvement). Excluding the eyes already blind at SFRT initiation, functional improvement was achieved in 7 out of 12 (58%) eyes, while none deteriorated. Acute side effects included local erythema in 5 and local alopecia in 11 patients. These findings resolved during the follow-up period. Endocrinologic evaluation revealed functional hyperprolactinemia in two and partial hypophyseal insufficiency in one patient. No other side-effects of SFRT were observed.

Several reports followed confirming these findings. BAUMERT et al. (2004) reported on a multiinstitutional experience on 23 eyes in 23 patients with pONSM. There were 4 males and 19 females. Indications for primary SFRT were tumour progression documented by imaging or symptoms (loss of vision, pain). Twenty-two patients had an ophthalmologically documented progressive visual deterioration. For two patients, treatment was recommended in order to prevent further growth of the tumour to the contralateral optic nerve. Seven patients had pain due to the meningioma and for six patients proptosis of the involved eye was an additional indication for treatment. Two patients had bilateral ONSM, of which only the symptomatic tumour site was treated. One patient was already blind in the affected eye for several years at the time of referral and one patient was nearly blind. Diagnosis was based mainly on diagnostic imaging and ophthalmologic examination, as histologic biopsies did not belong to the standard work-up due to the high risk of side-effects. All patients had CT and MRI scans of the orbit. All patients were immobilized and scanned using BrainLab relocatable stereotactic frame. All but two patients had an additional individually customized bite-block. BrainLab treatment planning system was used in all cases. GTV was the same as CTV, while PTV included a margin of 2–3 mm around the GTV (for the definition of the 95% isodose line). SFRT was delivered using three to five non-coplanar static fields, each conformed by MLC or individual cerrobend blocks. All treatment plans used one single isocentre. The dose was prescribed at the isocentre (ICRU 50). Total prescribed dose was 45–54 Gy in fractions of 1.8–2.0 Gy (median, 50.4 Gy) in 6 weeks. Patients were seen weekly during SFRT and 4–6 weeks after the last fraction. All patients underwent regular ophthalmologic control with examination of the visual fields and visual acuity. The first ophthalmologic and radiation oncology follow-up examination was performed 3 months after treatment. Thereafter patients were followed 6-monthly with clinical and ophthalmologic examination. Radiological examination included MRI at least once a year.

After a median follow-up of 20 months (range, 1–68 months), 16 (73%) out of 22 eyes with documented visual decrease before SFRT improved in vision, while 5 (22%) remained stable. One patient had continuous visual loss after SFRT. One patient deteriorated after 4 years, with stable vision. Visual improvement was documented for 13 patients already 1–3 months after SFRT. For three patients visual improvement was already subjectively reported during the SFRT and documented by ophthalmologic examination 3 months after SFRT. For eight patients visual improvement consisted of an increase in visual acuity of more than two Snellen lines; for one patient this was an improvement from light perception to hand motions. In the whole group visual acuity improved for 15 patients, visual fields for 8 patients. Visual acuity as well as visual field improvement was documented for seven patients. Visual fields showed no change in 11 patients. For three of seven patients having pain due to the tumour, the pain decreased during SFRT, for four patients 1–3 months after SFRT. One patient out of six with a proptosis experienced a decrease in proptosis, which was documented on imaging with a tumour decrease. On imaging, the tumour remained stable in almost all patients, one decreased and none increased in size. Regarding acute side-effects of SFRT, eight patients needed low dose steroids to decrease lip oedema during the SFRT. One patient suffered from increased pain for a short period of time after SFRT. Small areas of local hair loss at the end of SFRT were seen in all patients. Of late side-effects, one patient had increased headaches after SFRT. Regarding the patient with progressive visual loss, authors hypothesized that SFRT may have been administered too late. One patient developed a radiation retinopathy complicated by a vitreous haemorrhage and cataract 4 years after SFRT. In spite of vitrectomy, the visual acuity in that eye dropped to light perception.

An Australian study (RICHARDS et al. 2005) retrospectively reviewed a group of four patients (three women, and one man) with ONSM treated with SFRT. Mean age was 35 years (range, 26–51 years). They have been offered an SFRT after documenting progressive loss of visual acuity and/or optic nerve function and/or visual field. SFRT was administered with a mean dose of 43.5 Gy (range, 43.42–45 Gy) in a mean of 26 fractions (range, 25–27 fractions) using a frameless stereotactic system. The tumour target was imaged using both CT and MRI scans. The PTV covered CTV and an additional margin of at least 2 mm. The stereotactic system used circular collimators starting with 5 mm, 7 mm, 10 mm, and with increments of 2 mm up to 30 mm, with further increments of 5 mm up to 50 mm. Usually, a modification of a standard set of four non-coplanar arc fields were selected to provide homogenous isodose distribution. PTV coverage was with the 90% isodose line. At their most recent follow-up examination (2 years for three patients and 4 years for one patient), all patients had best corrected visual acuity of 6/12 or better and all patients retained visual acuity the same as or better than at the time of commencement of SFRT. All patients experienced improvement of optic nerve function measured by the degree of afferent pupil defect and/or red saturation and/or brightness saturation. Three patients had improvement of visual field following SFRT, but one patient developed field deterioration in the form of ring scotoma. In all four patients, disc swelling resolved leaving a pale, flat non-gliotic disc. No change in tumour size could be detected on MRI of any of the four patients. The most serious side-effect at the time of the report has been transient patchy radiation-induced hair loss in one patient. One patient has radiologically evident cerebral punctuate small vessel fallout in the field of irradiation.

Swiss study was provided by LANDERT et al. (2005). Seven eyes in seven patients underwent SFRT for pONSM documented clinically and radiologically (MRI). There were six females and one male with median age of 46 years (range, 27–66 years). Affected side includes the left eye in one patient and six patients with right sided tumours. There were two intraorbital, two intracanalicular and three intracranial ONSM. Indications for SFRT were deterioration of visual function with or without radiologically documented tumour growth. Patients have had a 20–40 or better visual acuity immediately before SFRT started. The median SFRT total dose was 54 Gy (range, 50–54 Gy) using daily fractions of 1.7–1.8 Gy over 6 weeks. Patients were immobilized and scanned in a relocatable stereotactic mask with integrated custom-made bite-block. GTV was defined as visible tumour on planning CT and was expanded by 3 mm three-dimensionally for the calculation of the PTV. Irradiation was performed with non-coplanar fixed beams conformed to the treatment volume. Baseline and follow-up assessments of visual acuity were performed as best-corrected visual acuity measured using Snellen charts and noted in a 20/20 ratio equivalent. Visual acuity was recorded at 3 months after SFRT in six of seven eyes and at the last follow-up visit in all seven eyes. The visual field was tested either by Goldmann kinetic perimetry or by automated static perimetry. A change in visual function was defined as change in visual acuity or visual field. The mean follow-up was 57 months (range, 21–142 months). The mean follow up after SFRT was 23 months (range, 8–40 months). Six patients experienced stable disease, while in one patient response was defined as stable-regressive, due to less

uptake of the contrast during the imaging. Six patients experienced improvement in visual function. Five eyes had an increase in visual acuity of three lines or more; one eye improved by one Snellen line. At 3 months after SFRT, visual acuity had improved in five out of the six eyes in which it was recorded. One eye lost two lines of visual acuity. Visual field improved in four patients, remained stable in two, and deteriorated in one patient. There were no long-term side-effects of SFRT. One patient had acute eyelid oedema and was treated with low-dose steroids with subsequent symptom resolution. In the same report, the authors presented the data on six untreated patients which were compared to the treated ones. There was a significantly better visual outcome for the treated group than the untreated group (p = 0.012).

Most recently, SITATHANEE et al. (2006) reported on their experience with SFRT in pONSM. There were 12 patients, 10 of whom were females and 2 were males, each with 1 eye involved Age ranged from 25 to 67 years (median, 41 years). Presenting symptoms included progressive visual loss (10 patients), proptosis (6 patients), facial numbness (2 patients), and impaired eye movement (1 patient). Of these 12 patients, 5 were initially treated with surgery after which they had no light perception. Indications for SFRT in these patients included residual tumour or tumour progression after surgery. Seven patients had their diagnosis made based mainly on imaging and ophthalmologic examination. Indications for SFRT in these seven patients were visual deterioration and proptosis with or without radiologically documented tumour growth. Visual acuities of these patients before starting SFRT ranged from 20/20 to 20/100 and six of them had impaired visual fields. SFRT was used in six patients, while stereotactic radiosurgery was used in a patient with a small tumour and no vision after surgery. Patients were immobilized and scanned in a relocatable Gill-Thomas-Cosman stereotactic frame. The number of isocentres used ranged from one to five. The mean average dose of SFRT was 55.7 Gy (range, 51.6–59.1 Gy), prescribed at 90% isodose, delivered in 1.8-Gy daily fractions over 5–6 weeks. Patients were followed at 1 month after completion of SFRT and then every 3–6 months thereafter. Ophthalmologic examination including measurement of visual acuity by Snellen lines and visual function measured by perimetry was performed. Follow-up MRIs were obtained at least once a year. Response to treatment was defined clinically by improvement of vision or presenting symptoms. After a median follow-up of 34 months (range, 7–66 months), there was no visual improvement in the five patients who had no light perception before SFRT. Among the remaining seven, four patients had improved visual acuity. Vision remained stable in two patients who had pretreatment VA 20/20 and 20/25. Four of six had improved visual function, and five of six decreased in proptosis. Follow-up imaging was available in six patients showing minimal tumour regression in five and stable in one patient. No tumour progression was observed. No serious acute side-effects were observed, perhaps due to oral steroids used in some patients. One patient had headache and temporary decreased vision for 4 months after SFRT and was fully recovered after steroid treatment. Visual acuity in that patient improved from 20/50 before SFRT to 20/25 at 52 month follow-up. One patient with uncontrolled diabetes and hypertension developed vitreous haemorrhage 2 years after SFRT. The visual acuity in that patient dropped from 20/100 to finger count and was not improved after vitrectomy. No visual deterioration of the contralateral eyes was observed.

Although one may object to the existence of only small studies and the occasional lack of prolonged follow-up in all presented patients, data from these studies enable us to draw some conclusions on the use of SFRT in pONSM. It is a uniform finding that relatively modest doses of radiation therapy, mostly ranging from 45 to 54 Gy and conventionally fractionated (mostly using 1.8 Gy per fraction), using the target volume typically expanding 3–5 mm from the known tumour margins, lead to at least 80% of visual improvement or stability, after the follow-up of several years. These results could have been better if cases with pre-treatment mild or moderate visual loss were represented more, since patients with marked improvement after SFRT are likely those having visual acuities ranging from 20/40 to 20/30, which may allow a greater potential for good treatment results, as reiterated recently by RICHARDS et al. (2005), LANDERT et al. (2005) and SITATHANEE et al. (2006). This is so for both visual acuity and visual fields where improvements are unprecedented with any other treatment modalities used historically in this patient population (Table 10.1). Importantly, these figures are observed as stable in the vast majority of cases after prolonged periods of follow-up.

Table 10.1. Studies using stereotactic fractionated radiation therapy in pONSM

Author	Year	No. pts	RT dose (Gy)	Functional outcome	Follow-up (median)	Side-effects
Liu et al.	2002	5	45–54 Gy	4 (80%) improvement; 1 (20%) stable	12–84 months (median 24 months)	No RON No RT-necrosis
Andrews et al.	2002	30	50.4 Gy	In 92% functioning eyes preservation of vision; in 42% improvement	2–71 months (median 22 months)	Visual loss (n = 2), Optic neuritis (n = 1) Transient orbital pain (n = 1) Total, 4 (13%)
Pitz and Becker	2002	15	54 Gy	100% improved or stable visual fields and visual acuity	Range 12–71 months (median 35.5 months)	No RON No RT-necrosis
Baumert et al.	2004	22	45–54 Gy	16 (73%) improved 5 (22%) stable	Range 1–68 mnthos (median, 20 months)	1 (5%) optic neuropathy and vitreous hemorrhage
Richards et al.	2005	4	43–45 Gy	100% improved/stable visual acuity 75% improvement in visual fields	Range, 2–4 yrs (median, 2 yrs)	Cerebral punctuate small Vessel fallout in RT field
Landert et al.	2005	7	50.4–54 Gy	85% improvement in visual acuity 86% improved/stable visual fields	Range, 8–40 months (mean, 23 months)	1 (14%) acute eye lid edema
Sitathanee et al.	2006	6	51.6–59.1 Gy	80% improved visual acuity 66% improved visual fields 83% improved proptosis	Range, 7–66 months (median, 34 months)	1 (16%) vitreous hemmorhage (in uncontrolled diabetes)

RT = radiation therapy; RON = radiation-induced optic neuritis

Interestingly, these results were coupled with an observation from all SFRT studies (Liu et al. 2002; Becker et al. 2002a; Pitz et al. 2002; Andrews et al. 2002; Baumert et al. 2004; Richards et al. 2005; Landert et al. 2006; Sitathanee et al. 2006) that functional improvements were not followed by significant and frequent decrease in tumour size on imaging done at various time points during the follow-up. This is in general agreement with earlier reports showing that RT rarely caused significant tumour shrinkage on imaging (Smith et al. 1981; Sarkies 1987; Kupersmith et al. 1987; Ito et al. 1988; Kennerdell et al. 1988; Dutton 1992; Turbin et al. 2002). Although that was a frequent reason for surgeons not to recommend RT in cases of rapid visual decline but to recommend surgery to immediately alleviate pressure to visual pathways (Schick et al. 2004; Roser et al. 2006), recent reports on the use of sophisticated techniques, other than SFRT, seems to confirm the observation of slow, if any, tumour shrinkage during and after RT (Eng et al. 1992; Lee et al. 1996; Klink et al. 1998; Grant and Cain 1998; Moyer et al. 2000; Narayan et al. 2003). It must, however, be clearly stated that improvement in visual function can occur even during the course of RT (Vagefi et al. 2006), as well as later on in the follow up period, and in neither case it was dependent on tumour shrinkage. It seems that an explanation, rather plausible, is that the main reason for this observation may actually be a combination of RT-induced oedema decrease and "decompression" of the functional nerve structures.

Contrasting these observations, a recent study of Henzel et al. (2006a) showed that there was a significant tumour volume reduction of meningiomas after stereotactic radiotherapy, albeit of the fact that none of 84 patients had pONSMs were included in that study. Nevertheless, in all cases the cavernous sinus had always been invaded. Using the stereotactic treatment planning system Voxelplan and the Novalis system (BrainLab), the treatment was delivered with a 6-MV linear accelerator using photons. Daily dose of 1.8–2.0 Gy was prescribed up to a cumulative median dose of 56 Gy (range, 50.4–60.0 Gy) Tumour volume shrinkage was quantitatively and three-dimensionally analyzed using the planning system. Mean tumour volume shrunk by 33% at 24 months and by 36% at 36 months after stereotactic RT. Younger age and smaller tumour volumes were determining factors, while there was no influence of prescribed dose, histology, sex, and previous operations. These results were reconfirmed in a larger series of the same group (Henzel et al. 2006b) where 100 out of 219 patients (46%) developed a regression while 117 patients (53%) were stable. Quantitative mean tumour volume shrinkage was 26.2% and 30.3% at 12 and 18 months

after SFRT, respectively. Five patients in this series had optic nerve meningioma involving the saggital sinus.

Another important finding further supporting SFRT as the emerging standard treatment of choice is very low toxicity observed in patients with pONSM treated with SFRT, which, in cases without significant extension outside the orbit is negligible. Toxicity in the study of Andrews et al. (2002) could be attributed to rather undisclosed predisposing factors and more extensive tumours in which planning was rather difficult, and accompanied with dose inhomogeneities leading to its occurrence. Also, there has been a recent report (Subramanian et al. 2004) of a case with radiation retinopathy occurring 2 years after SFRT (optic nerve dose, 54 Gy in 30 daily fractions; optic nerve head dose, 48–54 Gy; posterior retina dose, 27.8–48 Gy) for pONSM located intraorbitally and intracanaliculary did not provide additional information regarding this matter. Neither pretreatment factors that may have contribute to its occurrence nor the exact incidence of such findings among the other, presumably existing, cases of pONSM treated with either conventional RT or SFRT have been provided. It therefore remained unexplained why such patients developed retinopathy while still receiving 27–48 Gy to posterior retina. This has serious implications, as not to jeopardize the treatment success of SFRT, which effectively combined biological (fractionation; 45–54 Gy in daily fractions of mostly 1.8 Gy) and technological (stereotactic treatment planning, daily reproducibility of high precision, and high conformation of the dose to the desired treatment volume) aspects of treatment. This dose/fractionation was shown to produce *no* toxicity to optic nerve/chiasm when IMRT was used to treat irregularly shaped intracranial meningiomas other than that of the optic nerve sheath (Uy et al. 2002). These data fit into the data accumulated in the 2D era of radiation therapy which helped demystify RT-induced toxicity in these cases. It was observed that brain necrosis is extremely unusual after 54 Gy given in 1.8-Gy daily fractions, being 0.2% in an analysis, which included 1388 patients (Becker et al. 2002b). The risk of injury to the optic pathways also depends on the single and total RT doses. Without previous surgical damage to the pathways, with the single dose of < 2.0 Gy and the total dose ranging from 45 to 50 Gy, this risk was below 2% (Brada et al. 1993; Becker et al. 2002b). If the total dose increases to 54 Gy, the risk of optic neuropathy rises to roughly 5% (Goldsmith et al. 1992; Parsons et al. 1994). However, in the study on head and neck cancer (Parsons et al. 1994) with the dose of < 59 Gy no injury was observed in 106 optic nerves. With > 60 Gy, the 15-year actuarial risk of developing optic neuropathy was 47% with fraction sizes of >1.9 Gy, but was only 11% with fraction sizes < 1.9 Gy.

These findings have recently been reconfirmed by other authors. MILKER-ZABEL et al. (2005) reported on 317 patients with benign or atypical intracranial meningioma treated with SFRT. Six patients had optic nerve sheath meningiomas, none of which was resected, while in two patients biopsy was undertaken. All 317 patients were treated with a median dose of 57.6 Gy (range, 45–68 Gy) and a median daily fraction size of 1.8 Gy, five times a week. Unfortunately, no specifics were provided for the six patients harbouring ONSM. Nevertheless, stable disease was observed in 70% patients and reduction in 23% patients. As many as 43% percent of patients experienced an improvement in pre-existing neurologic deficits at the end of RT; 37% had reduction in diplopia, and 38% improvement in preexisting exophthalmos. Only 2.5% of patients developed new clinical symptoms without preexisting deficits, two of whom had reduced vision. No clinically significant acute or late grade 3 or greater side effects were observed. Although the results of this study may not instantly be valid for ONSM patients, due to there being only 6 cases, low toxicity in 317 patients, some of which received > 60 Gy, shows low toxic potential of SFRT even in cases where somewhat larger treated volumes were used.

CANDISH et al. (2006) reported on a series of 38 patients undergoing stereotactic RT for treatment of benign meningiomas. For treatment planning and delivery, patients were immobilized in relocatable stereotactic head frame (BrainLAB AG, Heimsteten, Germany) with associated bite-block, occipital impression, and facial Aquaplast. The median number of fields used was 6 (range, 4–10). Conformation by means of custom-made blocks in 9 cases and micromultileaf collimator in 27 cases. The median dose delivered was 50 Gy (range, 45–50.4 Gy) over 28 fractions. Clinical follow-up involved 6-monthly review and MRI until 2 years and then annual follow-up and imaging thereafter. Full endocrine and ophthalmic follow-up was mandatory in all patients. Six patients had optic nerve meningiomas, followed for a median of 28.5 months. Five patients have controlled their vision (three improved, two stable), while only one patient had a minor decrease in ipsilateral acuity with associated retinal changes compatible with RT at 58 months. MRI findings were stable with no evidence of progression of the primary tumour.

Similarly, the study of HAMM et al. (2006) reported on 183 patients with skull base meningiomas involving optic pathways, 8 patients having their tumours invading optic sheath. Unfortunately, although good results were followed by low toxicity, no separate analysis was provided for optic nerve sheath meningiomas.

Summarizing all available data from the literature, it is obvious that SFRT for pONSM is effective and low toxic treatment option. It is much more effective than any other treatment modality in this, largely unfavourable patient population presenting with existing visual loss. These results request consideration of RT in the treatment of pONSM early in the course of the disease. While surgery remains reserved for cases of large tumours causing blindness and preventing spread to intracranial sites, the only other treatment approach to be considered is observation. Unfortunately, observation is still practiced worldwide in expectation that some of pONSM will grow slowly and hence will lead to slow impairment of vision. At present, however, there are no tests allowing a precise prediction of growth velocity of an individual tumour. Furthermore, there is lack of clinical correlation between progression in imaging and progression in functional impairment. Finally, virtually all cases managed by observation end up in serious dysfunction or even blindness. This calls for a clinical assessment of ONSM patients combining both ophthalmologic examination and imaging (as each of these performed separately might miss signs of progression). As soon as either diagnostic tool shows progression, RT should be administered.

Taking into account the effectiveness of high-precision RT, the recent data call for change of the practice worldwide. Although prospective randomized trials investigating this issue are highly desirable, the rarity of this condition will probably prevent their performance in the near future. Therefore, evidence coming from available studies has to be considered, especially since RT seems the only treatment modality allowing stabilizing or even improvement of vision in patients with pONSM. Though a number of institutions are practicing this approach, there is no standard treatment approach worldwide. Hopefully, joint efforts of specialized centres capable of monitoring the disease and performing sophisticated RT will lead to a standardized protocol. Every effort should be made to spread awareness of these changes in treatment approach.

References

Adler JR Jr, Gibbs IC, Puataweepong P, Chang SD (2006) Visual field preservation after multisession cyberknife radiosurgery for perioptic lesions. Neurosurgery 59:244–254

Andrews DW, Faroozan R, Yang BP et al. (2002) Fractionated stereotactic radiotherapy for the treatment of optic nerve sheath meningiomas: preliminary observations of 33 optic nerves in 30 patients with historical comparison to observation with or without prior surgery. Neurosurgery 51:890–904

Arndt J (1993) Focused gamma radiation. The Gamma Knife. In: Phillips MH (ed) Physical aspects of stereotactic radiosurgery. Plenum Medical Book Company, New York, pp 87–128

Baumert BG, Villà S, Studer G, Mirimanoff R-O et al. (2004) Early improvements in vision after fractionated stereotactic radiotherapy for primary optic nerve sheath meningioma. Radiother Oncol 72:169–174

Becker G, Jeremic B, Pitz S et al. (2002a) Stereotactic fractionated radiotherapy in patients with optic nerve sheath meningioma. Int J Radiat Oncol Biol Phys 54:1422–1429

Becker G, Kocher M, Kortmann RD et al. (2002b) Radiation therapy in the multimodal treatment approach of pituitary adenoma. Strahlenther Onkol 178:173–186

Betti O, Munari C, Rosler R (1989) Stereotactic radiosurgery with the linear accelerator: treatment of arteriovenous malformations. Neurosurgery 24:311–321

Brada M, Rajan B, Traish D et al. (1993) The long-term efficacy of conservative surgery and radiotherapy in the control of pituitary adenomas. Clin Endocrinol 38:571–578

BrainLAB (2000) Radiotherapy solutions. User guide revision 4.2. Patient preparation

Brell M, Villà S, Teixidor P et al. (2006) Fractionated sterotactic radiotherapy in the treatment of exclusive cavernous sinus meningioma: functional outcome, local control, and tolerance. Surg Neurol 65:28–33

Candish C, Mckenzie M, Clark BG et al. (2006). Stereotactic fractionated radiotherapy for the treatment of benign meningiomas. Int J Radiat Oncol Biol Phys 66(Suppl):S3–S6

Das IJ, Downes MB, Corn BW, Curran WJ, Werner-Wasik M, Andrews DW (1996) Characteristics of a dedicated linear accelerator-based stereotactic radiosurgery-radiotherapy unit. Radiother Oncol 38:61–68

Duke-Elder S, Smith RJH (1962) The examination of the visual function. In: Duke-Elder S (ed) The foundation of ophthalmology: hereditary, pathology, diagnosis and therapeutics. System of ophthalmology, vol 7. CVG Mosby, St Louis, pp 370–374

Dutton JJ (1992) Optic nerve sheath meningioma. Surv Ophthalmol 37:167–183

Eng T, Albright N, Kuwahara G et al. (1992) Precision radiation therapy for optic nerve sheath meningiomas. Int J Radiat Oncol Biol Phys 22:1093–1098

Esterman B (1968) Grid for scoring visual fields. Arch Ophthalmol 79:400–406

Frankel KA, Phillips MH (1993) Charged particle method: protons and heavy particles. In: Phillips MH (ed) Physical aspects of stereotactic radiosurgery. Plenum Medical Books, New York, pp 43–85

Georg D, Bogner J, Dieckmann K et al. (2006) Is mask-based stereotactic head-and-neck fixation as precise as streotactic head fixation for precision radiotherapy? Int J Radiat Oncol Biol Phys 66(Suppl):S61–S66

Girkin CA, Comey CH, Lunsford LD, Goodman ML, Kline LB (1997) Radiation optic neuropathy after stereotactic radiosurgery. Ophthalmology 104:1634–1643

Goldsmith BJ, Rosenthal SA, Wara WM, Larson DA (1992) Optic neuropathy after irradiation of meningioma. Radiology 185:71–76

Grant W III, Cain RB (1998) Intensity modulated conformal therapy for intracranial lesions. Med Dosim 23:237–241

Hamm K-D, Henzel M, Gross MW et al. (2006) Stereotactic Radiotherapy of Meningiomas Compressing Optic Pathways. Int J Radiat Oncol Biol Phys 66(Suppl):S7–S12

Henzel M, Gross MW, Hamm K et al. (2006a) Significant tumor volume reduction of meningiomas after stereotactic radiotherapy: results of a prospective multicenter study. Neurosurgery 59:1188–1194

Henzel M, Gross MW, Hemm K et al. (2006b) Stereotactic radiotherapy of meningiomas. Symptomatology, acute and late toxicity. Strahlenther Onkol 182:382–388

Ito M, Ishizawa A, Miyaoka M, Sato K, Ishii S (1988) Intraorbital meningiomas. Surgical management and role of radiation therapy. Surg Neurol 29:448–453

Kennerdell JS, Maroon JC, Malton M, Warren FA (1988) The management of optic nerve sheath meningiomas. Am J Ophthalmol 106:450–457

Kjellberg RN, Preston WM (1961) The use of Bragg peak of a proton beam for intracerebral lesions. In: Second International Congress Series 36:E103

Klink DF, Miller NR, Williams J (1988) Preservation of residual vision 2 years after stereotactic radiosurgery for a presumed optic nerve sheath meningioma. J Neuro-Ophthalmol 18:117–120

Kondziolka D, Lunsford LD, Coffey RJ, Flickinger JC (1991) Stereotactic radiosurgery for meningiomas. J Neurosurg 74:552–559

Kondziolka D, Niranjan A, Lunsford LD, Flickinger JC (1999) Stereotactic radiosurgery for meningiomas. Neurosurg Clin N Am 10:317–325

Kooy HM, Dunbar SF, Tarbell J et al. (1994) Adaptation and verification of the relocatable Gill-Thomas-Cosman frame in stereotactic radiotherapy. Int J Radiat Oncol Biol Phys 30:685–691

Kortmann RD, Becker G, Perelmouter J, Buchgeister M, Meisner C, Bamberg M (1999) Geometric accuracy of field alignment in fractionated stereotactic conformal radiotherapy of brain tumors. Int J Radiat Oncol Biol Phys 43:921–926

Kupersmith MJ, Warren FA, Newall J, Ransohoff J (1987) Irradiation of meningiomas of the intracranial anterior visual pathway. Ann Neurol 21:131–137

Landert M, Baumert B, Bosch MM, Lutolf U, Landau K (2005) The visual impact of fractionated stereotactic conformal radiotherapy on seven eyes with optic nerve sheath meningiomas. J Neuro-Ophthalmol 25:86–91

Leber KA, Bergloff J, Langmann G, Mokry M, Schrottner O, Pendl G (1995) Radiation sensitivity of visual and oculomotor pathways. Stereotactic Funct Neurosurg 64:233–238

Leber KA, Bergloff J, Pendl G (1998) Dose-response tolerance of the visual pathways and cranial nerves of the cavernous sinus to stereotactic radiosurgery. J Neurosurg 88:43–50

Lee AG, Woo SY, Miller NR, Safran AB, Grant WH, Butler EB (1996) Improvement in visual function in an eye with a presumed optic nerve sheath meningioma after treatment with three-dimensional conformal irradiation therapy. J Neuro-Ophthalmol 16:247–251

Leksell L (1951) The stereotactic method of radiosurgery of the brain. Acta Chir Scand 102:316–319

Leksell L (1971) Stereotaxis and radiosurgery: an operative system. Charles C. Thomas, Springfield, IL, pp 5–52

Liu JK, Forman S, Hershewe GL, Moorthy CR, Benzil DL (2002) Optic nerve sheath meningiomas: visual improvement after stereotactic radiotherapy. Neurosurgery 50:950–957

Milker-Zabel S, Zabel A, Schultz-Elzner D et al. (2005) Fractionated stereotactic radiotherapy in patients with benign or atypical intracranial meningioma: long-term experience and prognostic factors. Int J Radiat Oncol Biol Phys 61:809–816

Miralbell R, Caro M, Weber DC et al. (2007) Stereotactic radiotherapy for ocular melanoma: initial experience using closed eyes for ocular target immobilization. Technol Cancer Res Treat 6:413–418

Moyer PD, Golnik KC, Breneman J (2000) Treatment of optic nerve sheath meningioma with three-dimensional conformal radiation. Am J Ophthalmol 129:694–696

Narayan S, Cornblath WT, Sandler HM et al. (2003) Preliminary visual outcomes after three-dimensional conformal ration therapy fort optic nerve sheath meningioma. Int J Radiat Oncol Biol Phys 56:537–543

Parsons JT, Bova FJ, Fitzgerald CR, Mendenhall WM, Million RR (1994) Radiation optic neuropathy after megavoltage external-beam irradiation: analysis of time-dose factors. Int J Radiat Oncol Biol Phys 30:755–763

Pitz S, Becker G, Schiefer U et al. (2002) Stereotactic fractionated irradiation of optic nerve sheath meningioma: a new treatment alternative. Br J Ophthalmol 86:1265–1268

Richards JC, Roden D, Harper CS (2005) Management of sight-threatening optic nerve sheath meningioma with fractionated stereotactic radiotherapy. Clin Exp Ophthalmol 33:137–141

Romanelli P, Wowra B, Muacevic A (2007) Multisession CyberKnife radiosurgery for optic nerve sheath meningiomas. Neurosurg Focus 23:E11, pp 1–6

Roser F, Nakamura M, Martini-Thomas R, Samii M, Tatagiba M (2006) The role of surgery in meningiomas involving the optic sheath. Clin Neurol Neurosurg 108:470–476

Sarkies NJC (1987) Optic nerve sheath meningioma: diagnostic features and therapeutic alternatives. Eye 1:597–602

Schick U, Dott U, Hassler W (2004) Surgical management of meningiomas involving the optic nerve sheath. J Neurosurg 10:951–959

Schlegel W, Pastyr O, Bortfeld T, Becker G, Schad L, Gademann G, Lorenz WJ (1992) Computer systems and mechanical tools for stereotactically guided conformation therapy with linear accelerators. Int J Radiat Oncol Biol Phys 24:781–787

Sitathanee C, Dhanachai M, Poonyathalang A, Tuntiyatorn L, Theerapancharoen S (2006) Stereotactic radiation therapy for optic nerve sheath meningioma: an experience at Ramathibodi hospital. J Med Assoc Thai 89:1665–1669

Smith JL, Vuksanovic MM, Yates BM, Bienfang DC (1981) Radiation therapy for primary optic nerve meningiomas. J Clin Neuro-ophthalmol 1:85–99

Solberg TD, Boedeker KL, Fogg R, Selch MT, DeSalles AA (2001) Dynamic arc radiosurgery field shaping: a comparison with static field conformal and noncoplanar circular arcs. Int J Radiat Oncol Biol Phys 49:1481–1491

Subramanian PS, Bressler NM, Miller NR (2004) Radiation retinopathy after fractionated stereotactic radiotherapy for optic nerve sheath meningioma. Ophthalmology 111:565–567

Tishler RB, Loeffler JS, Lunsford LD et al. (1993) Tolerance of cranial nerves of the cavernous sinus to radiosurgery. Int J Radiat Oncol Biol Phys 27:215–221

Turbin RE, Thompson CR, Kennerdell JS, Cockerham KP, Kupersmith MJ (2002) A long-term visual outcome comparison in patients with optic nerve sheath meningioma managed with observation, surgery, radiotherapy, or surgery and radiotherapy. Ophthalmology 109:890–899

Uy NW, Woo SY, Teh BS et al. (2002) Intensity-modulated radiation therapy (IMRT) for meningioma. Int J Radiat Oncol Biol Phys 53:1265–1270

Vagefi MR, Larson DA, Horton JC (2006) Optic nerve sheath meningioma: visual improvement during radiation treatment. Am J Ophthalmol 142:343–344

Villà S, Linero D, Marín S et al. (2000) Stereotactic fractionated radiotherapy (SFR) using three different relocatable frames". Poster workshop, proceedings 19 Annual ESTRO Meeting

Subject Index

List of Contributors

GREG BEDNARZ, MD
Department of Radiation Oncology
Thomas Jefferson University Hospital
111 South 11th Street
Philadelphia, PA 19107
USA

MARKUS BUCHGEISTER, MD
Klinik für Radioonkologie
Universität Tübingen
Hoppe-Seyler-Str. 3
72076 Tübingen
Germany

E. BRIAN BUTLER, MD
Radiation Oncology Department
The Methodist Hospital
6565 Fannin, DB1-077
Houston, TX 77030
USA

Email: EButler@tmhs.org

SAM T. CHAO, MD
Cleveland Clinic
Brain Tumor and Neuro-Oncology Center
Department of Radiation Oncology, Desk T28
9500 Euclid Avenue
Cleveland, OH 44195
USA

Email: chaos@ccf.org

JORGE OMAR HERNANDEZ, PhD
ABC Medical Center
Mexico City, Mexico
and
c/o The Methodist Hospital
6565 Fannin, AX121-B
Houston, TX 77030
USA

Email: omaovi@yahoo.com.mx

JOSE HINOJOSA, MD
ABC Medical Center
Mexico City, Mexico
and
c/o The Methodist Hospital
6565 Fannin, AX121-B
Houston, TX 77030
USA

Email: johingom@yahoo.com

BRANISLAV JEREMIĆ, MD, PhD
International Atomic Energy Agency
Wagramer Strasse 5
P.O. Box 100
1400 Vienna
Austria

Email: b.jeremic@iaea.org

JOHN S. KENNERDELL, MD
Chairman and Professor Emeritus
Allegheny General Hospital
320 East North Ave, Suite 116
Pittsburgh, PA 15212
USA

DOLORS LINERO, MD
Department of Radiation Oncology
Hospital Universitari Germans Trias. ICO Badalona
08916 Badalona. Barcelona
Spain

SIMON S. LO, MD
Associate Professor of Radiation Medicine
and Neurosurgery
Director of Residency in Radiation Oncology
Director of Neuro-Radiation Oncology and Stereotactic
Radiation Therapy
Department of Radiation Medicine, Arthur G. James
Cancer Hospital
Ohio State University Medical Center
300 West 1st Avenue, Ste 088a
Columbus, OH 43210
USA

Email: simon.lo@osumc.edu

MAHMOOD F. MAFEE, MD, FACR
Professor of Clinical Radiology
Vice Chair for Education
Residency Program Director
UCSD Medical Center
200 West Arbor Drive
San Diego, CA 92103
USA

Email: mmafee@ucsd.edu

JOHN H. NAHEEDY, MD
Chief Resident
Department of Radiology
University of California, San Diego
200 West Arbor Drive
San Diego, CA 92103
USA

ARNOLD C. PAULINO, MD
Radiation Oncology Department
The Methodist Hospital
6565 Fannin, DB1-077
Houston, TX 77030
USA

Email: apaulino@tmhs.org

FRANK PAULSEN, MD
Klinik für Radioonkologie
Universität Tübingen
Hoppe-Seyler-Str. 3
72076 Tübingen
Germany

Email: frank.paulsen@uni-tuebingen.de

SUSANNE PITZ, MD, PhD
University Eye Hospital
Langenbeckstrasse 1
55101 Mainz
Germany

Email: pitz@augen.klinik.uni-mainz.de

GUIDO REIFENBERGER, MD, PhD
Department of Neuropathology
Heinrich-Heine-University
Moorenstr. 5
40225 Düsseldorf
Germany

Email: reifenberger@med.uni-duesseldorf.de

MARKUS J. RIEMENSCHNEIDER, MD
Department of Neuropathology
Heinrich-Heine-University
Moorenstr. 5
40225 Duesseldorf
Germany

Email: M.J.Riemenschneider@gmx.de

JOHN H. SUH, MD
Cleveland Clinic
Brain Tumor and Neuro-Oncology Center
Department of Radiation Oncology, Desk T28
9500 Euclid Avenue
Cleveland, OH 44195
USA

Email: SUHJ@ccf.org

BIN S. TEH, MD
Radiation Oncology Department
The Methodist Hospital
6565 Fannin, DB1-077
Houston, TX 77030
USA

Email: bteh@tmhs.org

ROGER E. TURBIN, MD, FACS
Assistant Professor
Neuro-ophthalmology and Orbital Surgery
University of Medicine and Dentistry
New Jersey Medical School (UMDNJ-NJMS)
90 Bergen Street, Suite 6177
Newark, NJ 07103
USA

Email: turbinre@umdnj.edu

Salvador Villà, MD, PhD
Department of Radiation Oncology
Hospital Universitari Germans Trias. ICO Badalona
08916 Badalona. Barcelona
Spain

Email: svilla@iconcologia.net

Maria Werner-Wasik, MD
Associate Professor
Residency Program Director
Department of Radiation Oncology
Thomas Jefferson University Hospital
111 South 11th Street
Philadelphia, PA 19107
USA

Email: Maria.Werner-Wasik@jeffersonhospital.org

Helmut Wilhelm, MD, PhD
University Eye Hospital
Schleichstrasse 12-16
72016 Tübingen
Germany

Email:helmut.wilhelm@med.uni-tuebingen.de

MEDICAL RADIOLOGY   Diagnostic Imaging and Radiation Oncology
Titles in the series already published

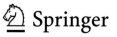
Springer

MEDICAL RADIOLOGY   Diagnostic Imaging and Radiation Oncology
Titles in the series already published

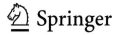

Springer